CAROL HENSEL'S AEROBIC DANCE & EXERCISE BOOK

Contemporary Books, Inc.
Chicago

Library of Congress Cataloging in Publication Data

Hensel, Carol.
    Carol Hensel's aerobic dance and exercise book.

    Includes index.
    1. Aerobic dancing.   I. Title.   II. Title: Aerobic
dance and exercise book.
RA781.15.H45   1983   646.7'5   83-7362
ISBN 0-8092-5538-3

**Photographs of Carol Hensel and Nancy Cobb (except where noted)
by Robert Holcepl and Don King.**

Published by Contemporary Books, Inc.
180 North Michigan Avenue, Chicago, Illinois 60601
Manufactured in the United States of America
Library of Congress Catalog Card Number: 83-7362
International Standard Book Number: 0-8092-5538-3

Published simultaneously in Canada by
Beaverbooks, Ltd.
150 Lesmill Road
Don Mills, Ontario M3B 2T5
Canada

Contents

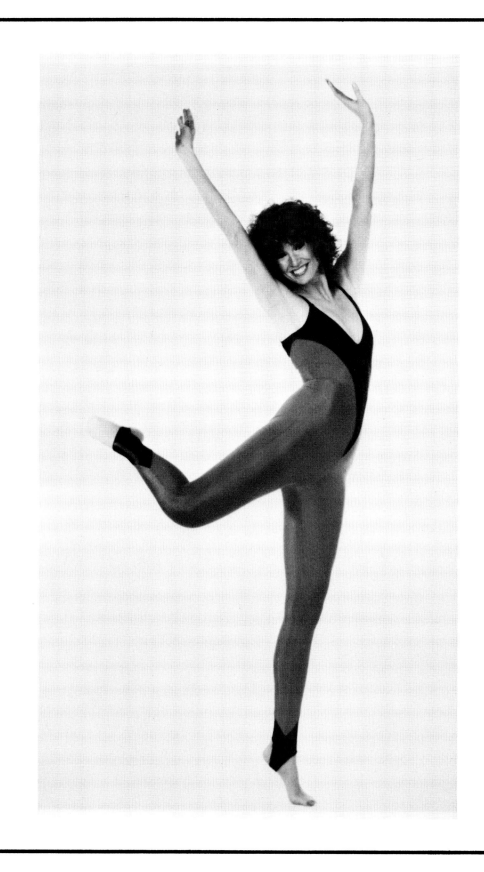

Introduction

I simply cannot imagine any other way to become physically fit than to dance and exercise to music. I have been moving to the beat since I was introduced to music by my parents at a very early age. I can remember how much my father enjoyed listening to classical pieces on the radio or record player. My mother was also a big music fan, with a greater appreciation for all types, including the rock and roll of the '50s.

Surrounded by music throughout my childhood, I gained a deep appreciation for its beauty and rhythm. While still a preschooler, I saw the ballet *Scheherazade.* To this day it is my favorite ballet because of its powerful music and the way foreign customs are reflected through dance.

I was very lucky to have had my own record player at that age. My father's records were off limits, but that didn't keep me from accumulating my own stack of 45s. Les Paul's guitar magic in "Jingle Bells" still makes me move when I think about it. I now know that a rec-ord player would be the first gift I would give my own children.

Later in life, when I began teaching a pre-school creative dance class, I used some children's dance records, available at that time only through special distributors. They were fun and gave the children the opportunity to play games like Choo-Choo Train, London Bridge, Musical Chairs, and Going through the Tunnel. But something seemed to be missing during these games, some part of the bubbling energy I saw whenever the children ran and jumped *before* class in their uniquely unin-hibited way. Even the kids who were terribly shy during my class were whooping it up while playing their own games. They simply were not as excited about playing organized games to music as they were when left to make up their own games.

I hit on the solution when I decided to bring in the records I had danced to as a child. When I was four I spent so much time with my little record player, dancing to tunes like "Purple

v

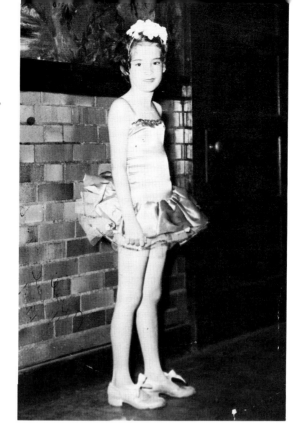

My first dance review, age six, at the Betty Adelman Dance Studio, Massilon, Ohio.

People Eater," "Splish Splash," and "Alley Cat," along with a stack of Walt Disney story songs, that an extra carpet had to be laid down in my dance area. There seemed to be hundreds of those upbeat rock and roll tunes from the '50s. My favorite tune from that era was "The Freeze," a song that quickly became the most popular in all the preschool dance classes I taught. It had a quick tempo and fun lyrics.

Watching preschoolers dance and play to these records made me realize that the music alone was enough to inspire exercise. The children were happier, more enthusiastic, and therefore livelier when left to their own reactions to music they liked. They simply didn't need the structured direction of the records I had originally tried.

Exercising to music has continued to be a successful way for me to teach people, whether children or adults, that they can have fun while exercising. Improving one's fitness level by learning new dance movements and techniques set to popular music instills a natural state of euphoria that is addictive. Once you have felt the wonderful "high" brought on by a good workout, you will stay with it as long as it is convenient and fun to do so.

In my *Aerobic Dance and Exercise Book*

you will discover how exercise, body awareness, and dance can work together to form a self-improvement system that makes you feel and look better. Most of us have a tendency to be lazy and can easily find excuses for not exercising. With this book, the right music, and the convenience of matching my aerobic dance and exercise program to your busy schedule, you'll have no excuse for not exercising at least three times a week. None!

The program I have organized for this book will teach you all the basic dance steps and movements you will need for a complete workout. Also included are warm-ups and stretches for loosening your muscles and joints and cooldown routines that stress relaxing and tapering off from the rigorous exercise program. The program is most effective as a calorie burner and body toner as well as being an excellent form of aerobic conditioning. I have noted those specific areas of the body (hips, thighs, stomach, etc.) that benefit most from particular exercises. That way you can concentrate on problem areas of the body, and incorporate them into a personalized workout, if desired.

Within two or three weeks you'll begin noticing a difference in how you feel. Your arms and legs will look better than ever as your muscles become firmer, longer, and leaner. As you continue your fitness program on a regular basis you'll start to notice a host of additional benefits:

- Increased energy and stamina
- Positive feeling about yourself
- Greater ability to handle stress and tensions
- Loss of weight
- Loss of inches
- Improvement in sleep
- Reduction in total food intake
- Better circulation
- Increased flexibility, coordination, body control, rhythm, and dancing ability

One of the nicest benefits of my program is that you can use it anytime, anywhere—in the privacy of your home or with friends or neighbors—without having to be tied down by inconvenient class schedules.

As you get into my aerobic dance and exercise program you'll quickly realize that exercising does not have to be drudgery, done only for end results. It can be fun. Just give your body the chance to swing and dance freely and naturally to music. Don't worry about landing on the correct foot or applying all the suggested techniques. By taking this approach, you'll discover that dancing offers much more than you ever imagined!

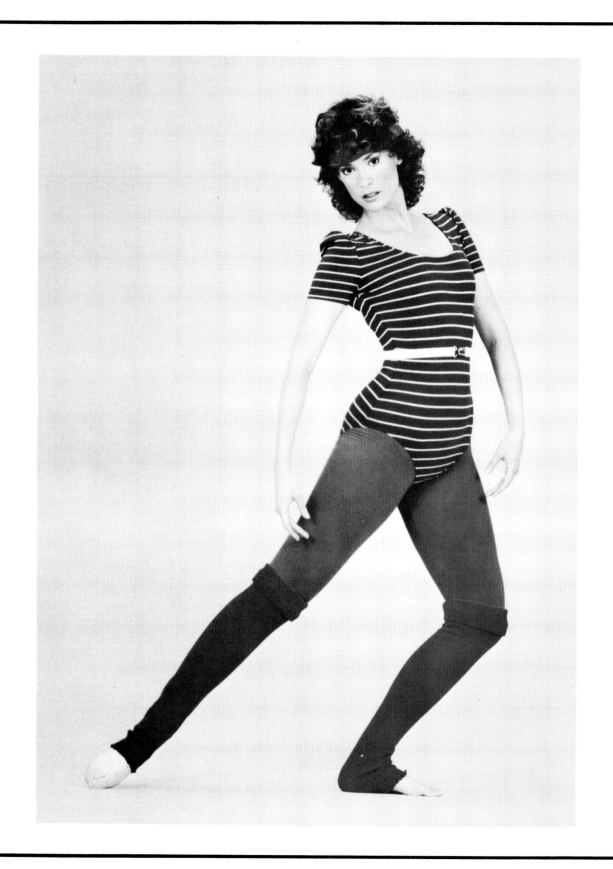

1

Why Exercise?

Your body depends on oxygen to exist. Oxygen is taken from the air you breathe and transported to the body tissues by way of the blood vessels. The capillaries are the terminal ends of the arteries and carry the oxygen in the blood to the cellular structure of the body tissues. Your very existence depends on the health of your blood vessels. To maintain the circulation of oxygen-carrying blood through your vessels you must have a healthy heart.

As you age, your blood vessels change, becoming less elastic due to deposits of cholesterol and other products of metabolism on the vessel walls. When the blood vessels become so filled with these deposits, blood will not travel through them, and the tissues of the body will not get an adequate oxygen supply, causing them to function poorly. Diet and exercise help maintain healthy blood vessels. Occasionally speeding up the flow of blood through exercise helps to preserve the integrity of the blood vessels.

Diet control alone will not be enough to maintain a healthy body, nor will exercise alone suffice. Many people do more physical work than is necessary to stay healthy but are actually fat from overeating. Others eat an excellent diet but are so sedentary that, even though they are within their weight limits, they suffer from premature cardiovascular disease.

Adequate regular exercise will make you feel better. The increased circulation that results from a period of exercise increases the output of the endocrine glands and body enzymes. A person who gets adequate exercise is rarely constipated. The deep breathing caused by exercise aids in preserving healthy lungs. There are millions of people who have not had enough exercise in years to cause them to take a deep breath. Imagine lungs that are never expanded by the deep breathing demanded by exercise!

Who should exercise? Everyone should exercise, except those suffering from an incapacitating illness. Some people with illnesses or handicaps may, however, benefit from a

1

planned exercise program. Former president Franklin D. Roosevelt, who was an invalid from polio and could not stand, exercised daily. He was persistent in exercising the parts of his body that he could move and control. He kept his body and mind active for his whole life, even during four consecutive terms as President of the United States. Considering his serious health problem, his record of achievement was outstanding. Undoubtedly his exercise routine aided his efforts.

You must tailor your exercise regimen to the condition of your health and take a sensible approach. Common sense dictates that your approach to exercise depends on your current physical condition. A healthy lumberjack can go full blast into an exercise program, while a sedentary bookkeeper must gradually work into the program.

Even age is no deterrent to sensible forms of exercise. The aged must be careful about twisting, for bones that are osteoporotic may fracture when joints are twisted. Your bones will be healthier and able to tolerate exercise at an older age if you have exercised throughout life.

When my great-grandfather was over 90 years old he ran four miles to work and did farm chores when he returned home in the evening, after he had jogged back another four miles. And just as no one is too young to learn, no one is too young to exercise. In fact, young children seem to be exercising continuously while awake. Try to follow a four-year-old around.

To get an idea of how exercise increases awareness, self-assurance, and euphoria, visit a YMCA or YWCA gym at the conclusion of a group game such as volleyball. You will notice that everyone is noisy, jubilant, excited, and happy. I have noticed this over and over. After a period of exercise healthy people feel great, even if fatigued.

The impression an individual makes on others depends on the whole person. Body movements, posture, facial expressions, and stride are traits that contribute to your total image. Why exercise? Regular exercise in adequate amounts can enhance many of these factors, which contribute not only to your image but also to your general sense of well-being.

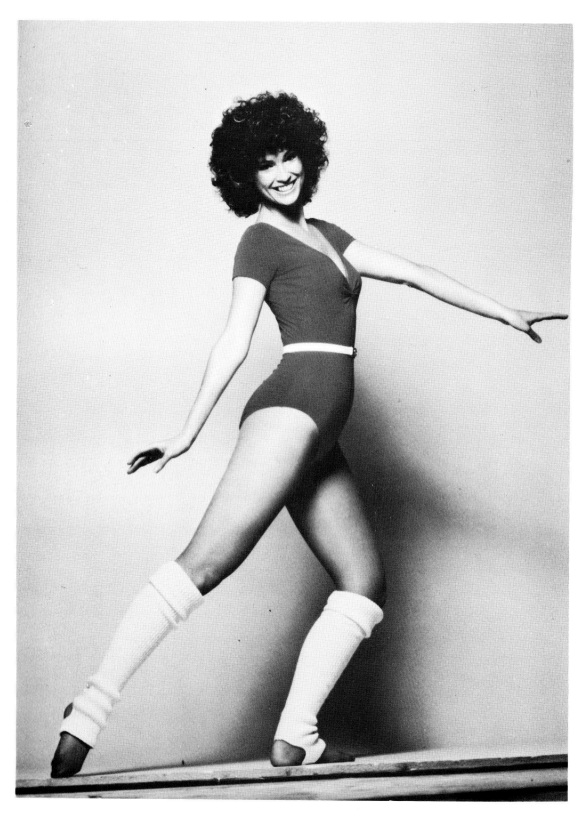

Photo by Bill Pappas

2

The Fitness Frame of Mind

You now know why you should exercise. But is this enough to convince you to do so? For many of us it is not. You may find that your attitudes—conscious and subconscious—get in the way of your best intentions. In this chapter is a brief review of two basic ways you can begin to adopt a fitness frame of mind: behavior modification and exposure of those myths and excuses concerning exercise that often stand in your way.

BEHAVIOR MODIFICATION

Through the use of behavior modification you can learn to change your poor health habits into new lifestyle activities that include proper exercise and diet.

Behavior modification simply means the learning of new habits through the use of constructive reinforcement and rewards. Pavlov made it famous with his salivating dogs, which would be fed after a dinner bell had been rung, until eventually just the sound of the bell would make them drool.

We use behavior modification all the time when we teach our pets tricks. A pat on the head does wonders for a dog who is learning to shake hands. This is positive reinforcement. Negative reinforcement is useful in its own way. House training a dog is seldom accomplished without a swat or two.

Understanding behavior modification begins with understanding your subconscious. This is the behavioral area that seems to function on its own with little or no input from your conscious or active mind. If you are like me, doing the dishes requires next to no concentration. I'm usually miles away while my hands are deep in the suds. The same goes for glancing through the junk mail, which seems to grow every day. Folding clothes is another example of robotlike behavior. Before you know it everything is organized in neat little piles. But where was your mind? Was it thinking about last night's Scrabble word that somehow eluded you? Hopefully you soon will include proper exercise and diet in your list of subconscious activities.

Subconscious cues are the signals that tell you to put the folded jeans in the jeans pile, clean your plate even though you feel full halfway through the meal, and jump into the car to go three blocks instead of walking. You pay no attention to this type of signal because it is a part of a mental process you are not conscious of. You must learn to recognize these subconscious cues, especially the negative ones.

Your emotions have their own set of reactions. How often do you just lie around feeling sorry for yourself or bored and then follow it up with a trip to the fridge? As children, many of us received special sweets when we were sick, a practice that we often continue for ourselves after we have grown up. Feeling lonely or sad is often compensated for with a piece of cake or, worse, two pieces of cake. The satisfaction gained by eating sweets is immediate. Blood sugar goes up and we feel temporarily boosted. The taste buds are jumping for joy and our troubles may be momentarily forgotten. But 10 minutes after we've eaten the harmful food we're back to feeling lazy and blue, and our subconscious is signaling for more. The vicious cycle begins.

Certain times of the day seem to trigger unhealthy subconscious reactions. Once the habit of eating has been formed, it's hard to break. Breakfast, lunch, and dinner are the big ones, but many of us have the mid-morning snack, the afternoon snack, the late evening snack, and finally the bedtime snack.

Understanding these subconscious cues is the first step to changing them. Negative subconscious cues can be made positive by altering your responses to them. A whole new set of responses is offered to you through a change to physical well-being. Examining all your subconscious reactions is difficult at first; some may find it beneficial to keep a running log of eating habits and excuses for not doing something else instead of snacking.

You must examine exactly how you feel when you are eating but are not hungry and when you are just lying around doing nothing.

What is taking place? How long is it going on? What are you eating? What are you doing? Where is all of this happening? If you analyze your negative reaction from every angle, you will soon recognize its cause, and that's the first step to changing it. If you let these bad cues occur whenever they feel like it, you're enabling them to dominate your behavior. They won't change by themselves, they won't go away, and, worst of all, they aren't even recognized for what they are by most people. Now that you know how your subconscious cues came to be, you can change them or eliminate them entirely.

The key to behavior modification is recognizing bad cues and changing or eliminating them. Think through an average day in your mind and pick out a certain behavior you wish to change. Jot it down, if you wish. Recognize that you are in command. You shape your subconscious. Every time you become aware of a bad cue dictating your response, you must eliminate it and replace it with behavior that is positive, beneficial, and self-satisfying.

These three steps of behavior modification—elimination, replacement, and reinforcement—should be taken for every negative subconscious response you uncover. It may be a little difficult at first—discovering the bad habit, stopping it, replacing it, and finally patting yourself on the back—but with practice all these steps happen in a wink. Finally, they don't happen at all because the new habit becomes your new reality.

After you've eliminated the response to the bad cue, you must substitute a new positive response for it. In many cases these new responses can be temporary because healthy positive responses to unhealthy negative cues tend to erase the bad cues altogether.

We've all heard the term *positive reinforcement* concerning the teaching of children. It's the same thing you do to yourself when you alter your own behavior. The natural contented feeling you get when you know that you are doing something right is one of the strongest feelings humans can have. Every bouncing step you take with your new healthy body is a positive reinforcement. Your mind is glowing with the knowledge that you're taking care of your body, adding energy to your life, and assuming a positive outlook. The increased awareness you gain from examining your subconscious puts you more in tune with your real self, your real needs, and your real capabilities.

Confidence and stamina will grow in all your physical activities. Being in sound physical shape gives your mind and body the ability to respond quickly and positively. Waking more refreshed from less sleep and sleeping more soundly is another benefit of a healthy body. Dreary chores seem less of a duty because they now take less time. Your spare-time hobbies and activities become more enjoyable. In fact, everything becomes more enjoyable now that you really enjoy yourself. There is no better reinforcement in the world than a healthy, happy body and mind.

Compliments from your friends on your new body should boost your ego a bit, but don't worry when they start tapering off. People will get tired of complimenting you on the same thing. Let your own self-esteem be the driving force behind your positive reinforcement. Self-respect and personal pride are the greatest measures of your success. These are the feelings that will pull you through the tough times, and there will be some of those.

It seems that within any exercise program there comes a time when your progress seems to stop. Even though you are continuing in the program as you always have been, nothing seems to be happening. If you're a woman, this may be caused by an unusual water weight buildup, but it is more likely the natural result of your body's settling into your new physique. It happens periodically in all exercise and diet programs and shouldn't be taken as a sign of failure. The body is not a statue of granite that can be evenly whittled down the same amount every day. It is a living, flowing organism with its own internal clocks and schedules. Take

heart, even though results may not be evident in the form of pounds falling off and inches vanishing away; if you stay on your program, you'll see the results rolling in again after a couple of weeks. Occasionally, depending on the person, it can last as long as a couple of months. Don't get discouraged. This stage, where results level off and don't change, is called a *plateau*.

During these plateaus your positive reinforcements have to be at their best. I've seen discouragement creep into an otherwise positive attitude and peck away until the old bad habits are taken up again. Now that you know that plateaus are the normal readjustments of your body during any weight loss program, you can remain confident that positive results will start up again. The tape measure is a more reliable measuring device than the scales as you monitor your success during my exercise program. How your clothes fit is the best indication of all.

Water retention during menstrual periods may even add weight and inches to your body, especially if you've reached a plateau. It's a common experience that is easily recognized and understood, so you shouldn't worry about it.

Another excellent way to reward yourself is by using role models for positive reinforcement. The more you become like one of your favorite movie stars, athletes, or entertainers, the more you will admire yourself. Enjoy those second glances you're now getting; you deserve them.

Diet control is discussed elsewhere, so I won't dwell on it here. But as far as your attitude about food goes, your new diet need not be thought of as a restraining tactic, like some kind of protective shield in front of your mouth. The healthy foods that are available to replace the fattening ones are many and varied.

Snacking is so ingrained in our culture that it is one of the most difficult negative subconscious cues to seek out and replace. Just say, "No thanks, I'm full," to those pushy hostesses or visiting aunts who love to tempt you with sweets and starches that are nutritional zeros. Healthy snacks range from fresh vegetables to cheese, from fruits to peanut butter, and almost any refrigerator has one or more of these. The harder outsiders try to tempt you, the greater the indication of your success, and that is a wonderful reinforcement by itself.

My exercise and dance program is designed as a complete program and should be followed from warm-up to cool-down. But that doesn't mean that you can't take out individual routines and use them as positive responses to negative cues. Many times the best response to those subconscious junk food cues is a 10-minute walk. After you learn my warm-up exercises you'll find them easy to do at times of behavior modification. You will find that an exercise break is often much more effective than a nap when you're attacked by the "blahs" in the middle of a project. Fatigue can be fought off by the increased rate of blood circulation and the released muscle tension brought about by exercise. Exercise is one of the greatest responses you can give to negative subconscious cues, and a healthy, good-looking body is one of the best reinforcements there is against the blues.

Behavior modification is the most successful technique for sustaining your new positive mind, healthy outlook, and active body. Old bad habits have been completely removed and replaced by a new way of life full of self-respect and pride. Using behavior modification keeps your muscles toned and the excess weight off.

EXERCISE MYTHS AND EXCUSES

Dispelling the Myths

Strenuous Workouts Should Be Preceded by Big Meals

False. There is nothing you could do to jeopardize your workout more. After eating, your body is busy breaking down the food into suitable forms for digestion. Eating immediately prior to working out can cause you to tire easily. You will not have the same vitality and vigor with which to exercise when you feel full. The same energy depletion can result even from eating a small meal or snacking before a workout.

I remember one strict ballet instructor at a workshop who would not allow us to eat or drink anything except small amounts of water during our breaks. Now I understand why. Sometimes drinking a lot of liquids before exercising can bring on abdominal cramping during a dance routine—cramping that will not recede until after a rest. By stopping you put a damper on achieving aerobic endurance. If you must have something in your stomach—especially when taking an early morning class—a meal of orange juice and a raw egg in a blender with fresh fruit is very nutritious and not too heavy to digest.

Vitamins Give Extra Energy

Wrong. Vitamins, when used as a dietary supplement, can be beneficial to your general health, but there is no evidence from controlled studies to suggest that any great benefit in energy gains can be derived from taking large amounts of vitamin C or E or multiple B-complex vitamins. You cannot depend on vitamins alone. Most of your dietary needs should be filled by a well-balanced diet.

There are two types of vitamins—water-soluble and fat-soluble. The fat-soluble vitamins are A, D, E, and K. It is generally accepted that ingesting any of these particular vitamins over the daily requirements can cause excessive storage and possible toxicity. Water-soluble vitamins, such as C and B-complex, are not stored and may need to be replaced. If a person eats too many processed foods, there is a strong possibility of becoming deficient in these vitamins.

Concerning vitamins' energy-giving property, evidence is accumulating that C and B-complex vitamins do help people "feel" better, leading to a sense of well-being. A diet in which all the food groups are represented, however, helps prevent vitamin deficiencies.

Workout Preparation Calls for Filling Up with Water or Salt Tablets

Not necessarily. When you initially begin working out you may lose an excessive amount of salt, but once you begin to get into shape and become better conditioned there will be a marked decline in the amount of salt lost through perspiration. As far as drinking those commercial drinks containing salt, water, glucose, and other little goodies is concerned, they are basically harmless but unnecessary. The best guideline for water regulation is to drink when you are thirsty.

"Quick Energy" Foods Help during Workouts

Not true. Your body has ample stores of glycogens (your body's storehouse of carbohydrates) to provide energy for those working muscles. The concept of "quick energy" foods just has no logical basis, even though the practice has been propagated for years. Carbohydrate foods can have a major effect on your performance in sports in which sustained physical activity is maintained over a long period of time. But unless you are an Olympic contender or a professional dancer getting ready to work out for a four-hour stretch, you do not need these simple carbohydrates.

Exposing the Excuses

"I'm Too Fat to Work Out"

I cannot think of a better way to remain fat for a lifetime than to sit in a chair in front of TV reruns and say, "I am just too heavy to exercise," or "It's too late to start now." Nobody is asking the extremely obese person to go out and run the Boston Marathon. But there is

no reason in the world why a little exercise, and I do emphasize *little* at first, along with a controlled weight reduction diet (see a doctor), cannot be the first step toward a healthier and, in all likelihood, much happier person. Besides, it is much easier to stay on a diet when using an exercise program. Not only are you stabilizing your metabolism; you are also still burning off calories after exercising. The workout can help decrease your appetite.

As with anyone else, the overweight person in particular should try not to rush too fast into an exercise program. Many times I have seen people get excited and work so hard on their newfound discipline of strict diet and daily exercise that they lose fat only to put it back on just as fast. This is an unrealistic approach. If it's not something you can live with for a lifetime, then you will only be trapped in a "yo-yo" syndrome.

Everyone's favorite routine is from my first album. The exercises are a combination of swinging sit-ups and leg stretches, done to the tune of "I Will Survive." The routine is seven minutes long. The first time you survive the full seven minutes you'll have a great feeling of achievement. That is a better feeling than you can get from any box of doughnuts!

"I'm Too Old to Exercise"

I have wished for a long time that more retirement homes, nursing homes, and other places where many senior citizens can be found would initiate some form of aerobics program. Exercise keeps the body as well as the mind young. Many of the physical problems of aging can be managed successfully by modern medicine. Much too often the elderly suffer instead from a melancholic form of depression. They will benefit not only physically from exercise but psychologically as well. Joining an exercise group can be a great social outlet, a chance to make new friends. This, along with the effects of exercise on physical well-being and self-awareness, can help improve their mental attitude, bringing on a kind of rejuvenation. When I was a swimming instructor one of my best friends conducted a senior citizens' aqua exercise program. I served as lifeguard while she taught. I enjoyed watching the class grow from a small group to one of our most popular classes. It renewed my faith in the fact that in aging you can still grow, learn, and improve as a person.

Many seniors preferred water aerobic exercises to those on land because of the therapeutic benefits. It was easier to withstand jogging in place in the water than to endure the jarring effects of jogging on land. Many postmenopausal women frequently suffer from osteoporosis. This is a calcium deficiency of the bones that increases the risk of bone fractures. The water acted as a cushion due to its buoyancy.

This is also good for severe cases of arthritis.

Instead of using the jogging and hopping aerobic dance steps designated for land, I suggest that senior citizens walk through the steps just using arm movements. Remember, the objective of aerobic exercise is to work with enough intensity and rhythmic duration to achieve a training effect. This can be done without jogging or hopping, which is why an aerobic dance program is especially good for those who think they're too old to exercise.

"I Don't Have the Time"

In the time it takes to sit down and watch your favorite TV rerun, you could be taking the time to add years to your life. It's very simple: take the time now or lose the time later.

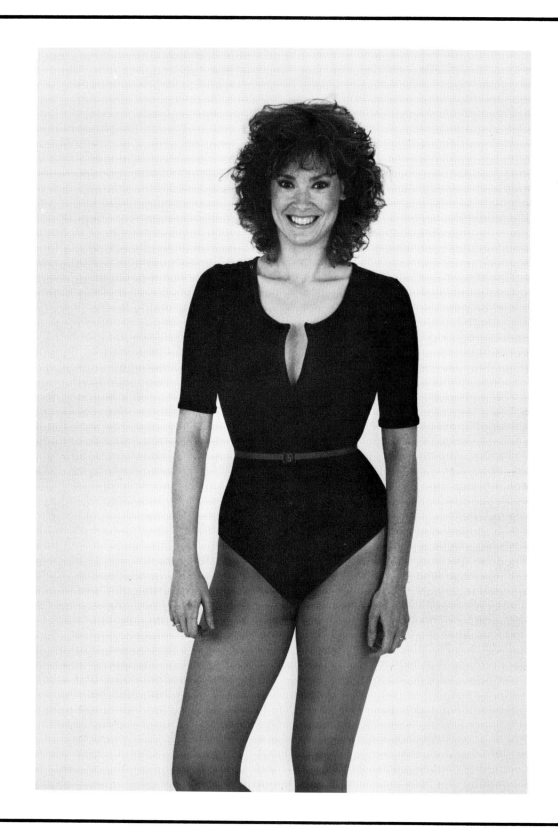

3

The Importance of Nutrition

No book on exercise and physical fitness should be written without stressing the need for good nutrition. Exercise and what you eat are not exclusive of one another. In fact, good nutrition and good exercise must balance each other out. You cannot have one without the other. Your body is an extremely complex machine, one that has very definite fuel requirements to run efficiently. You would not expect to get into your car, push the gas pedal, and move down the driveway if the fuel tank were empty or if you filled up with Dr. Pepper the last time you hit the service station. Likewise, you should not place undue demands and expectations on your body without first making certain that its nutritional needs are met. The correct amount and type of fuel are vital to your body!

Men and women have told me many times that they have had difficulty completing exercise programs because they were becoming fatigued. In many cases they appeared to be healthy and in good shape physically, and many had been following a formal exercise program for some time. What I usually found, after asking a question or two concerning their diets, was an obvious answer to their fatigue problems. They were simply not eating right. If you plan to derive full benefit from a fitness program, your body must receive the correct nutrients—correct in amount as well as in variety.

There is a very distinct correlation between energy levels required for exercise and the amount and type of fuel you deliver to your body. Indulging in fad diets would, in many cases, deny your body what it needs to maintain the energy levels called for in prolonged exercise. That does not necessarily mean that the more you work out, the more food you have to eat. The idea that the greater the amount of exercise, the more calories you need is a myth. It simply means that when you eat you should eat with nutritional sense.

NUTRITION VERSUS DIETING

Just the other day I was browsing in the local bookstore, and I could not believe the number of books, magazines, and pamphlets on the shelves pertaining to diets, health, and beauty. By the time I managed to read through all of them I would be ready for a nice retirement home. Diet after published diet promised that a person could stay thin forever. Fad diets promised the hope of becoming thinner, healthier, more attractive, and therefore happier. In an attempt to find the "new, slimmer, trimmer you," hopeful readers quickly hop from one best-selling diet to the next. The fact that there are so many varied diets on the market should make it obvious that they cannot all be right. First of all, no strict diet should be initiated without first consulting a doctor.

In defense of some very talented and well-meaning individuals, some diets offer a well-rounded balance of nutritional requirements, and some are merely foolish. But many could prove quite harmful to the person who is out for a quick "fix." Some diets are like those get-rich-quick schemes—great on promise, not so great on substance.

All too often, if you follow a fad diet, chances are that after a couple weeks of obeying all the rules and strictures of the diet so diligently you will decide to "cheat" and eat something that even Henry VIII would not have indulged in. All the binge does is negate any work you have already put into the diet. Dieting is not something to do between episodes of overeating. Nutritional dieting is a way of life. You can try every newfangled, promise-them-the-world diet that comes on the market, looking for that secret recipe, that miracle formula, but the solution will inevitably be a sensible diet along with an ongoing fitness program.

Crash dieting and exercise (or crash exercising and dieting) are not conducive to good health. In most cases a good exercise program must include a balance of nutritional dieting and exercise. (In some cases an exercise program may have to be preceded by a controlled weight-reducing diet for those who are extremely overweight. Consult your physician.)

NUTRIENTS—YOU ARE WHAT YOU EAT

For a long time nutritionists have been aware of the fact that to ensure good nutrition no single food pattern should be adhered to. People do not require specific foods; we require specific nutrients. In other words, it's not so much what we eat but what is *in* what we eat. If you want to live a long and healthy life, it's important to take care in what you put into your stomach. Mankind has made some remarkable progress in the last 30 years. Unfortunately, however, along with the advent of the golden arches and little cream-filled cakes wrapped in cellophane came the decline of the nutritional diet. Americans now eat more fats and more sugar (on the average) than a body needs in three lifetimes.

Since you have probably long forgotten what you learned in your high school health classes, I'll refresh your memory as to the main nutrients, how they are important to good health and exercise, and some common sense rules to follow about the foods you eat.

What Are Nutrients?

Every time you open your mouth to eat something you are in all likelihood partaking of a nutrient in one form or another. There are basically three nutrients we garner energy from: proteins, carbohydrates, and fats. They are all important. Each has its own function within the body, yet each interacts with the others. Unfortunately, some so-called diets exclude certain nutrients altogether, which could be detrimental to the dieter.

Proteins

Many people think protein usually comes in the form of a big, juicy, broiled filet mignon covered in mushrooms. Most of us were taught that meat and potatoes are the way to go, but today we know that vegetables are another source of protein. Some experts believe that plant life may actually be a much healthier source. Since all of the essential parts of protein cannot be found in any one vegetable, however, the safest course probably would be a healthy combination of both animal and plant foods. Further, beef and other red meats are not the only animal sources of protein. In addition to pork, lamb, and veal, we can turn to fish and poultry, which offer protein with less fat.

The building blocks of proteins are the amino acids. Your body just won't work without them. A diet that lacked amino acids would cause severe nausea, dizziness, low blood count, low blood pressure, insensitivity to touch, loss of hearing, impaired equilibrium, and eventually death. Not a pleasant prospect.

To get down to facts, there are 23 amino acids, 14 of which are produced within your own body. The other nine must be obtained through food on a daily basis. I cannot stress enough the importance of amino acids in your diet. In fact, the nine that the body receives from food are called the *essential amino acids*. They are essential because without them your body will not be able to manufacture the other 14. If even one of the essential aminos is missing from your diet, it could conceivably throw off your whole metabolism.

Very few foods contain all the essential amino acids. Some foods that do contain all nine are lean red meats, milk, and cheeses. Almonds are another source of complete protein, but you would have to devour so many that it would be impractical. You do not want to overdo it on meats and cheeses either, because of the fat content. A well-balanced diet of all the protein groups is your best bet.

A note to vegetarians: I am not a strong advocate of vegetarianism, but I can appreciate the fact that many people have chosen a meatless diet as a way of life. As I stated before, most vegetables do not contain all the proteins necessary to a good, nutritional diet, though it is possible to obtain the essentials through a combination of vegetables, legumes, and grains. To be on the safe side, an octo-lacto-vegetarian diet—one that is rich in natural cheeses and eggs—is probably the best. Amino acid concentrates are also available on the market for purists who do not wish to eat any animal products.

Carbohydrates

When your body wants or needs energy it will usually look to carbohydrates to supply the fuel. Carbohydrates are the body's main source of fuel. Carbohydrates come from plants. In a sense all animal life on earth relies on plant life to survive. Plants produce carbohydrates, animals eat plants, ruminants such as sheep and cattle convert the carbohydrates in the plants to protein, and mankind eats the animals (as well as the plants).

Carbohydrates are the starches and sugars in your diet. The body, amazing machine that it is, breaks down the carbohydrates into simple sugars such as glucose. Glucose is so important that we cannot survive without it. It is the free sugar floating in the bloodstream, supplying fuel to the brain, which takes care of the rest of your complex body. As in most nutrients, what the body cannot use for energy will often stay in the body in the form of fatty tissue.

Carbohydrates can be broken down into two main groups: simple carbohydrates, or simple sugars; and complex carbohydrates, such as starch and cellulose. The simple sugar sources are fruit sugars, corn syrup, honey, and that tasty little treat, sucrose, which is commonly known as *table sugar*. Each American now consumes between 100 and 130 pounds of sugar a year, on the average! While I am on the subject I might as well take some time to interject some thoughts on table sugar. I use very little sugar, a habit that I suggest everyone follow. Besides being devoid of almost any nutritional qualities, it is considered a contributing cause of tooth decay, heart disease, obesity, and other ailments.

Some people believe that eating foods that are high in simple sugar content will give them that extra boost or increase stamina during workouts. They are only fooling themselves. When the guy on TV extolls the virtues of chomping down on a candy bar between meals for that needed pickup in the afternoon he is being basically truthful. It will give you a quick burst of energy, but it will burn itself out just as quickly. What happens is that the pancreas will begin manufacturing extra insulin due to an increase in the blood sugar level. When this happens the body reacts by causing a severe drop in the blood sugar level. Instead of feeling exhilarated and full of energy you will tend to feel fatigued, with a large appetite to match. When you should be working out you are heading to the fridge instead. Stay away from those "quick energy" sugars.

Since the body needs carbohydrates, it is best to try the complex carbohydrates, which are less refined and take longer to metabolize. Thus they supply the body with energy over a more sustained period of time. Your body will function much better if you are not constantly jolting its systems. Examples of complex carbohydrates are cereal grains (wheat, oats, corn, and rice), potatoes, peas, beans, many fruits and vegetables, and tapioca.

Another example of complex carbohydrates is cellulose (stems and skins from many fruits and vegetables). Cellulose is a highly fibrous carbohydrate that cannot easily be digested but supplies the body with the roughage it needs to process solid wastes through and out of the body.

Fats

Fats, like proteins and carbohydrates, are an important energy source. The body needs some fat in the diet to function properly, to supply the body with fatty acids essential for healthy skin and proper body growth. Fat deposits in

the body prevent heat loss through the skin and act as a cushion for vital organs. The problem with fat is that most Americans consume much more fat than is needed by the body. Fat is a more concentrated energy source as it supplies the body with more than twice the amount of calories per gram than do proteins and carbohydrates (one gram of fat supplies nine calories, while carbohydrates and proteins each supply only four). Obviously, a diet high in fats will add much to the caloric level of the body, and what the body does not burn off or use, the body keeps in the form of fat deposits. The same holds true for the other nutrients—all extra unburned calories are stored in the body as fat. That is exactly why exercise is so important as a supplement to a good diet.

The best way to limit calories in your diet, if you wish to control or lose weight, is to reduce consumption of high-fat foods. Stay away from the saturated fats—butter, margarine, lard, and salad oils—and stick to the polyunsaturated fats such as vegetable and corn oils as much as possible. While the saturated fats may be as much as 80–90 percent fat, there are much less obvious sources of fat in our diets. Foods such as choice or prime steaks, mayonnaise, nuts (pecans, walnuts, almonds, and macadamia nuts have a fat content of 50–80 percent), meats, and some poultry are at least 10 percent fat. Chicken has a fat content of less than 1 percent as long as the skin is removed and the chicken isn't fried, while broiled steaks and chops are as high in fat as 50 percent. Many medical authorities believe that fat in your diet can lead to an increased cholesterol level in the blood, which has been linked to heart disease.

Fiber

Fiber is not truly a nutrient, but it should be an important part of everyone's diet. Unfortunately, in recent years American dietary trends have greatly reduced the amount of fiber our bodies receive. With increased consumption of processed foods, meats, and poultry, along with a decrease in the amounts of fresh fruits and vegetables, we have been consuming less fiber. The only source of fiber in our diets comes from plant life. Processing usually eliminates the fiber from whole grains (wheat, in particular), and meat and poultry provide no fiber. Recently, many weight-reducing diets have extolled the virtues of high-fiber diets, mainly in the form of raw fruits and vegetables and unrefined cereal grains. As long as the diet is balanced, this is not a bad idea. Because of their bulk you can usually feel full without consuming a meal the size of a family Thanksgiving dinner. Fibrous foods are also generally low in calories.

The importance of fiber in your diet has become increasingly recognized as it remains an important focal point for nutritionalists. Already studies have suggested a correlation between fiber consumption and a lower incidence of many diseases prevalent in the large intestine and possibly a reduction in blood cholesterol levels, a leading cause of atherosclerosis (fat-clogged arteries). If nothing else, fiber promotes regularity.

SUMMARY

We have just covered the three main nutrients. These are the nutrients that supply energy to the body. You really cannot function without all three as a constant part of your diet. But when not consumed in balance, or if your diet consists of more than your body can use, you are asking for trouble. Remember, what the body does not use for energy is stored in the form of fatty tissue. The key to good health is a nutritionally sound diet complemented by a constant and enjoyable exercise program.

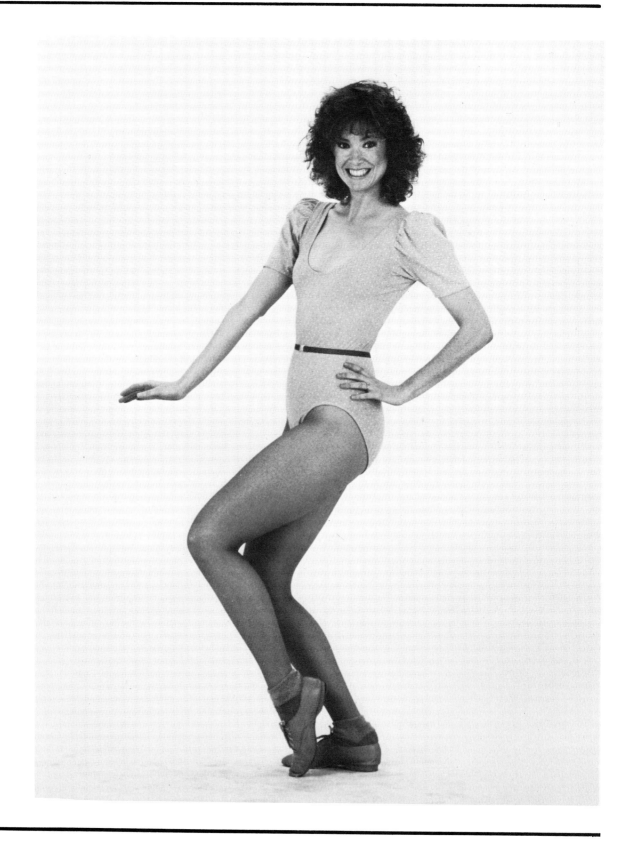

4

Exercising Aerobically

Aerobic dance is an innovative method of exercising that promotes cardiovascular fitness in enjoyable yet effective ways. This program combines expressive dancelike routines with a challenging regimen of aerobic exercises that increase the strength and endurance of your heart, lungs, and circulatory system.

The word *cardiovascular* pertains to the heart and the blood vessels that carry the oxygen in the blood throughout your body. The heart is a muscular organ whose basic function is to pump oxygen-rich blood to the tissues. Exercises that cause a sustained increase in the heart's activity and in oxygen consumption are therefore referred to as *aerobic*. The word *aerobic* comes from the Greek words *aer,* meaning air, and *bios,* meaning life.

By increasing your pulse rate for an extended period of time, aerobic exercises enhance cardiovascular fitness and stamina. Additionally, these exercises burn calories faster and with less fatigue than other forms of exercise. Although exercise alone is not the most effective way to lose weight, aerobic dance programs along with healthy dieting shrink the size of fat tissues while toning up the muscle tissues.

The benefits of aerobic dance are many. As your circulatory system gains strength you'll notice a definite decrease in appetite. Calories even continue to burn off at twice the normal rate up to five hours after the workout is over. Another benefit of aerobic dance workouts is the complete toning of all the body's muscles. Every muscle is exercised, not just a certain few, creating an overall healthy body. Increased physical stamina comes quickly after you have followed an aerobic dance program for a month or so. You'll find yourself ready to start that second tennis match. Also, because of your healthier circulation, your complexion improves, giving you that glow so noticeable in healthy people. The greatest benefit from a healthy body is the self-satisfaction you feel from the good things you have done for yourself. (More on aerobic dance's benefits can be found later in this chapter.)

THE TARGET HEART RATE

The effectiveness of a cardiovascular exercise program can be measured by gauging your pulse and comparing it with your target heart rate, which is the rate at which your heart should be beating during a sustained exercise program. A supervised treadmill test is the most accurate way to find your target heart rate, but you can find it yourself quite effectively. Start with the number 220 and subtract your age. This gives you your maximum heart rate. Take 75 percent of that figure to give you your approximate target heart rate for exercising. For example, if you are 30 years old your maximum heart rate is 190 and your target heart rate is 142.5.

The following chart is a general guide to approximate target heart rates according to age:

Age	Maximum Heart Rate	Target Heart Rate
20	200	150
25	195	146
30	190	142
35	185	139
40	180	135
45	175	131
50	170	127
55	165	124
60	160	120
65	155	116

After a month you may have lowered your target heart rate by as much as 20 beats per minute. This is an excellent measuring system for your increasing rate of endurance. After your target heart rate has fallen off somewhat, try to see if you can get it back up to where it was when you first started exercising by putting a little more oomph into your workouts.

Just as important as it is to reach your target heart rate, it is vital not to exceed it. If you exceed 85 percent of your maximum you are exercising too vigorously and should slow down.

If you are tiring easily, yet exercising within your target heart rate range, reassess your range and lower it. Maintain a pace at which you still work hard but do not overextend yourself. How do you know when you are above or below your target rate? Simple. Take a break during your exercise program to measure your pulse. Place two fingers lightly over the artery near the center of the inside wrist or at the carotid artery located on either side of the neck. Don't press down too hard or you'll impede the blood flow. Using a stopwatch or second hand of a wristwatch, count the number of beats for a period of 15 seconds. Multiply this number by four to get your heart rate in beats per minute.

POINTERS ON FOLLOWING THE PROGRAM

Aerobics works. Just get started. But, as the slogan says, "Think safety first." If you are over 35 or have had any health problems whatsoever, it is advisable to consult a physician before undertaking this or any other exercise program. If you wish, an EKG test may also be performed. Even if you're under 35, if you haven't had a physical examination in the last year you should have one before you start out. Pregnant women should always see a doctor.

Start the exercise program gradually, evenly, and with common sense. Patience will reward you soon enough, and in three to four weeks you will be conditioned enough to participate easily in the most strenuous routines. Listen to your body. It will tell you how to pace yourself properly.

Try to wait at least an hour and a half after eating before starting to exercise. If you have ever had a cramp, you know why it's wise to wait. I know many people, including myself, who exercise in the morning, therefore eliminating that problem.

Wearing comfortable footwear such as tennis shoes is a good idea whenever you are doing the hopping or jumping routines in my aerobic dance program. Good all-purpose sneakers serve as a cushion against injuries to your feet and knees. Clothes should be loose-fitting and comfortable. Shorts and T-shirts are just fine. Some women might prefer the extra support provided by leotards and support tights.

A wooden floor is the best area to work out on, but if that isn't available a carpeted floor is good. Watch out for those really thick carpets, though; they have been known to trip up even the most experienced exercisers.

The routines in my aerobic dance and exercise program are designed with varying degrees of difficulty. I don't mean that it is actually difficult to learn the routines. In fact, even the least experienced dancers can easily learn the steps, and the amount of sophisticated style you put into the exercises really is unimportant. What I mean about degrees of difficulty is intensity—the actual strengthening work you put into a particular routine.

Each routine can be walked through with your arms down if you're at the beginner stage. The hopping or jumping that's called for in certain dance steps is optional. You may walk through these particular routines, if you wish. This is a good way to slow down your exercise pace and heart rate to suit your own endurance level.

If you are in good shape, you can do all the routines normally. You can even add more hopping and jumping steps to many of the exercises. A couple of examples are replacing the knee lifts with knee hops and jumping while you do the hip twists. You can be as creative as you want when you learn to mold these routines to your particular strength.

You may soon be hopping and jumping all over these routines. But remember to land evenly on the bottom of your feet, not way up on the balls of your feet or way back on the heels. Shin splints and pulled Achilles tendons may result if you improperly land on your feet over and over. Whichever way you decide to work out with these routines, remember to keep moving. Muscles must be cooled down after a vigorous exercise session, just as they must be properly warmed up.

I recommend that you work out at least three times a week for 30–45 minutes to begin with, in order to maintain aerobic endurance, muscle flexibility, and body awareness. This does not mean exercising on three consecutive days and then laying off the next four. The best beginning program is to exercise on alternate days, such as Tuesday, Thursday, and Saturday. As you progress and begin feeling more fit you'll want to increase both the number of days and the length of exercise time.

To improve your level of aerobic fitness you need to push your heart rate up to its maximum working level for 15–20 minutes. Each workout should begin with at least 10 minutes of warm-up and stretching and end with the same amount of cool-down routines. Plan on spending at least 35 minutes on the entire workout. Do not skimp on any of these three areas because each is of vital importance.

The manner in which you breathe while exercising directly affects the nature of your movements, both internally and externally. As a beginner you might have a tendency to hold your breath while placing total concentration on performing the movements correctly. It's important to remember *not* to hold your breath since it will rob you of energy as well as lessen your ability to move with ease and strength.

The proper technique for breathing is to inhale when you need maximum power for the movement and exhale when your body is releasing. You will discover that you generally inhale when stretching, reaching, lifting, or raising your body and exhale when you bend or bring your limbs close to the body.

WHY AEROBIC DANCING?

As I stated, aerobic exercises can come in many forms. I chose dancing. Why? The answer is simple. I wanted an exercise program that could benefit me in a multitude of ways, and I wanted to be able to enjoy it at the same time. The choice was easy—aerobic dancing. First of all, I could work out at home—no more trying to find the time—or money—to run down to the spa. I also love to dance to music, and aerobic dance is the most self-expressive form of exercise I know.

What makes aerobic dancing so effective is that it is not drudgery. Many people view exercise only as a means to an end. They start a program for all the right reasons, then become bored with it and eventually drop out. Aerobic dancing is such a fun way to become fit that you can almost forget that you're working out because at the same time you are enjoying yourself.

THE BENEFITS OF AEROBIC DANCE

The benefits of aerobic dance are many. Some are interrelated, some are more obvious than others, but let me assure you that not long after you begin the program you will see the definite benefits that can be derived from aerobic dancing. In addition, you will feel the effectiveness of aerobics at work within your body which carries over into many other aspects of your life, such as leading you to a better body awareness.

Other benefits of aerobic dancing are as follows:

- It strengthens the entire cardiovascular system, improving the heart's pumping efficiency. This enables the heart to pump larger quantities of blood with each stroke, improving oxygen transmission to all parts of the body.
- It improves muscle tone throughout the body. This improves the general circulation of the body, thereby lessening the work load placed on the heart. In aerobic dance every muscle is exercised.
- Aerobic dancing improves the entire circulation system. Oxygen-rich blood travels more rapidly and efficiently to your muscles, vital organs, and skin. This better blood supply contributes to a healthier complexion, as mentioned earlier.
- It strengthens the respiratory system, eliciting improved air flow in and out of the lungs. You will breathe better.
- Due to increased oxygen demands over a sustained period of time, your body's systems will begin to work more efficiently. This will give you more daily energy. Instead of having that fatigued feeling all the time, you will be able to engage in physical activities over a longer period of time without becoming tired or running out of breath. With this increased physical stamina, within a month or so you'll find yourself ready and willing to take a walk after work instead of collapsing on the couch, play 18 holes of golf instead of nine, and so on.
- In aerobic dance calories continue to burn off at twice the normal rate even up to five hours after the workout is over. After an aerobic exercise session you can sit down, pick up a book, and relax and still burn off more calories than you normally would while resting.
- Due to high energy demands during workouts, aerobic dancing can burn off more calories faster and with less fatigue than other forms of exercise. You may be able to burn off as many calories by jogging, cycling, or swimming, but time and weather demands are minimized in aerobic dancing. You can burn approximately 300 calories in a moderate 45-minute dance class.
- Aerobic dancing can help control your eating habits. Due to the blood circulation demands made on your body during aerobic workouts, your desire for food is diminished. You simply don't feel like eating. The fact that your body continues to burn calories after you have completed your workout, however, should not be a reason to eat more or to indulge in snacking.
- Aerobic dance can help you achieve better body posture and carriage. When muscles that enable you to stand, walk, and sit correctly are properly exercised and trained, you move better. This puts less strain on the back muscles and you suffer less fatigue.

- Aerobic dancing can aid you in losing weight and trimming your body by losing inches.
- Aerobic dancing can be done just about anywhere—a fitness program you can take along even when you travel.

- You can develop increased flexibility, balance, body control, and coordination through aerobic dance. These improved physical abilities will carry over into other sports and activities.

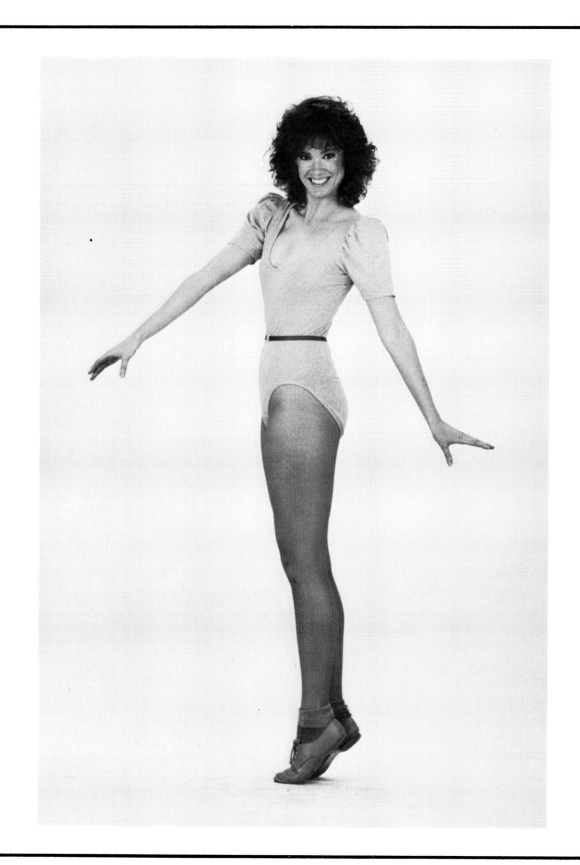

5

Warming Up

Warm-up routines are the most important part of any exercise program. Neglecting the warm-up phase can make you more apt to pull or strain a muscle. This is especially true for beginners who are not accustomed to regular exercise. Even the fittest of the fit must warm up to prevent an unwanted injury.

The warm-up routines are the slowest and most elementary of all my dance routines. Beginners can use these exercises for the first few workouts. Then they can gradually build onto each workout to form a new and more strenuous routine. This way, beginners are not putting a sudden, overwhelming demand on poorly toned or tense muscles.

Frustration and exhaustion can result from rushing into my dance and exercise program too quickly. It's hard to stay with any program that is too demanding at first. The typical American starts and ends a few different diet and exercise programs several times each year. This causes the yo-yo syndrome. No one can afford to fall into that on again, off again rut

that often ends in failure.

The warm-up routines are my favorites. To warm up I like to use music that has a flowing melody and an upbeat rhythm. Most of us have a tendency to be lazy, so I like to use music that motivates.

I am often asked, "What is the best time of day to exercise?" I like to turn the music on first thing in the morning, before I give myself a chance to make excuses. It's a great way to start the day, relaxing and allowing your muscles to feel the energy of the music. Remember, you're home alone, so feel totally free and uninhibited. Doing your routines in the morning also gives you the opportunity to use all the energy you've stored up from the previous night's sleep. You just need to get started. You will become refreshed and wide awake.

The warm-up will tune your body up for the lively aerobic routines that follow. The exercises in the warm-up phase prepare the muscles by making them more pliable and flexible. The warm-up exercises also raise the body temperature enough so it is less likely for you to become injured.

I'd like to say a few words about soreness here. The soreness you feel when exercising for the first time is normal. Don't worry too much about this. It will gradually taper off in about three days. Don't totally stop your program because of soreness after the first workout. Give yourself a day's rest without exercise, then slowly stretch the sore muscles, gently repeating the same exercise that most likely caused you the soreness. A hot bath or shower does wonders after working out, relaxing, and soothing tense and sore muscles.

Most soreness can be eliminated by remembering to do the all-important warm-up routine, no matter what particular type of aerobic activity you choose to do for that day.

I've had so many friends ask me what they might have done to injure themselves while playing racquetball, softball, basketball, and the like, and my first question to them is, "Did you warm up?" Their answer is always, "Well, uh, no, I didn't." Remember, no matter how much fun you are having while you are playing a sport, you are still making big demands on poorly toned and stiff muscles if you haven't warmed up properly.

I remember learning the hard way. I was 14 years old, cheerleading at a basketball game, when I finally overdid it. Being young and impatient, I never warmed up and got away without injury for years. I was doing what I considered a fairly easy routine, going down into a full split, when for some crazy reason I twisted my body the wrong way and pulled ligaments in my lower back. For years that injury bothered me. It was only after I was forced to warm up and stretch properly many times a day while teaching my own classes that my lower back pain finally disappeared. At any age, the warm-up is the most important stage of any exercise program.

STRETCHING FOR FLEXIBILITY

Flexibility and stretching go hand in hand. When joints bend and straighten, muscles expand and contract. It's the muscles that take the most abuse when you stretch beyond your limits.

Built into each muscle is a nerve system called the *stretch reflex*. As the extended muscle reaches its limit, the stretch reflex signals the muscle to contract, making the muscle tighten up if you try to stretch it further. Stretching past this point tears the muscle fiber, causing the formation of scar tissue and the pain of an overextended muscle.

There is no need to feel pain to increase your flexibility. If you're hurting, something is wrong. Slight soreness can be expected when you are introducing exercise to long unused muscles, but not pain.

The warm-up routines from my aerobic dance program include side stretches and forward bends that loosen up your muscles and eliminate stiffness before you do more strenuous exercises.

Never bounce while stretching. Bouncing fools the stretch reflexes into tightening up your muscles each time you bounce.

To become more flexible you must make stretching a part of your daily life. You should try to do a little stretching every day. But remember to do the proper warming up exercises first. Do your stretching exercises gently, gradually, and comfortably.

The flexibility you obtain from stretching exercises is quite beneficial. It helps you move freely and gracefully. You become more in touch with your body as you relieve stress. Flexibility also reduces your chances of muscle strain as it increases your ability to take part in everyday active sports. The loosening of tight muscles helps them become lean and trim instead of loose and bulky.

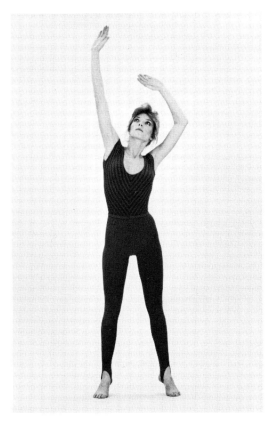

Reach right.

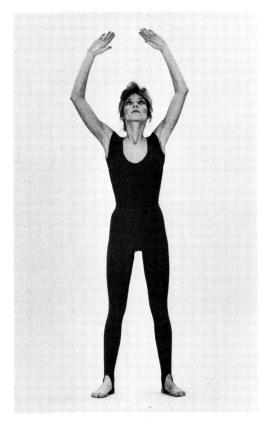

Back to the original position.

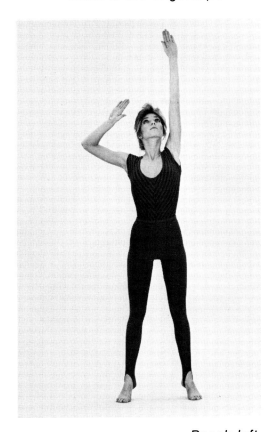

Reach left.

REACH

Start with arms relaxed overhead, feet apart, and heels on the floor. Reach up, lifting the heels and stretching first with the right arm. Drop the heels and relax the arms, returning to the original position. Reach up again, lifting the heels and stretching next with the left arm. Repeat the movement, alternating right and left arms.

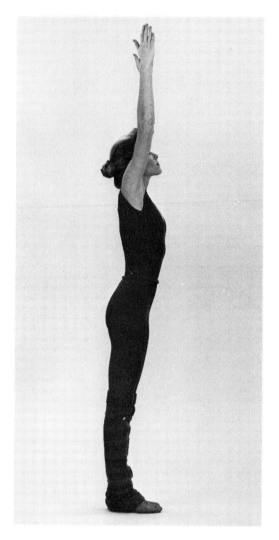

Starting position.

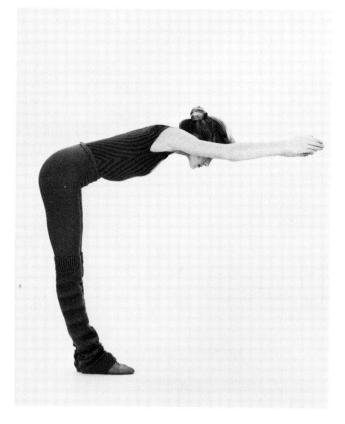

Bend forward.

BACK STRETCH

Start with arms straight overhead and feet together, stretching up the rib cage through to the fingertips. Release the torso forward and relax the arms down to the side. Continue bending down. Finish with the head and arms down and relaxed. Do not try to touch toes. Return to the original position and repeat.

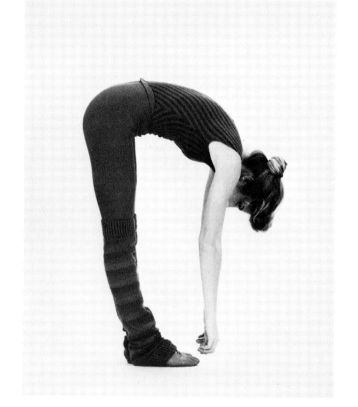

Down and relax.

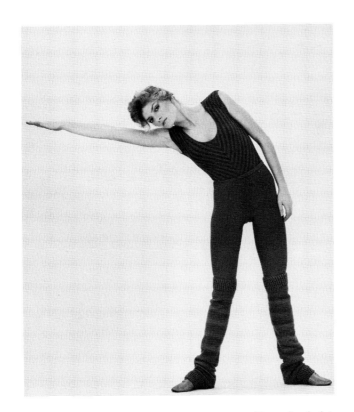

Reach right.

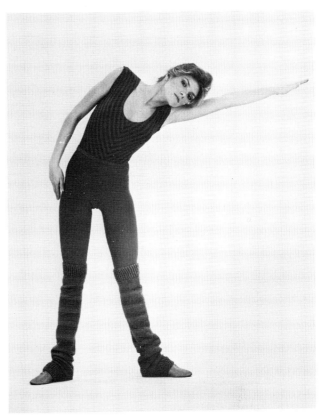

Reach left.

SIDE REACH

Start with feet apart, heels flat on the floor, and arms at your side. Extend the right arm and reach to the side. Then move to the left and extend the left arm. Continue, alternating sides.

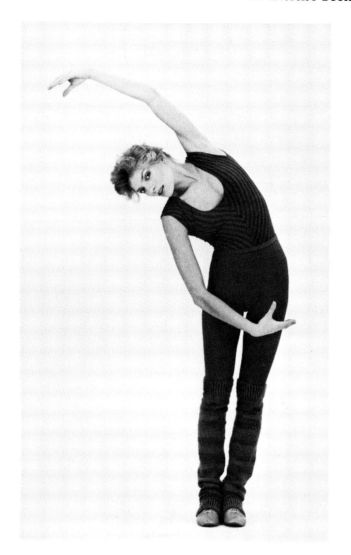

Stretch right.

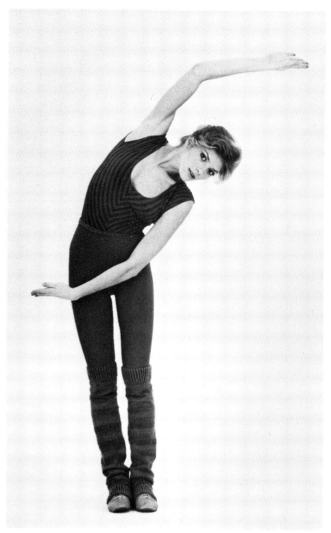

Stretch left.

SIDE STRETCH

Start with feet close together. Reach the left
arm overhead and stretch to the right with
the right arm down in front of the body. Then
stretch to the left with the right arm overhead
and the left arm in front. Swing the arms
back while dropping forward. Finish the
movement by lifting the arm up over the head
and stretching.

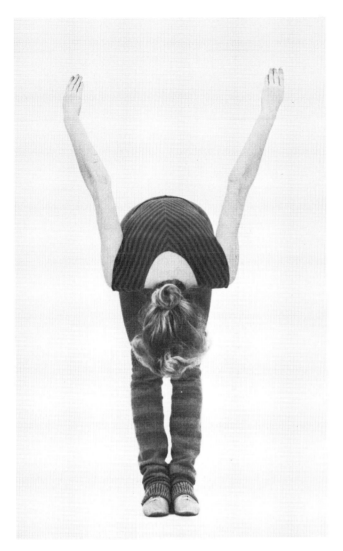

Drop forward.

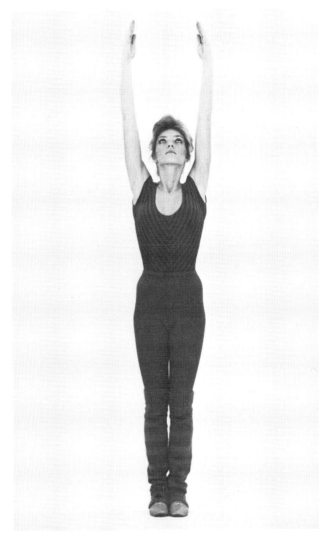

Stretch up.

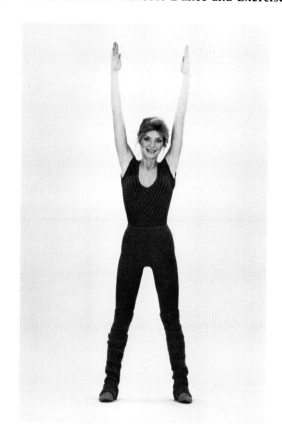

Arms overhead.

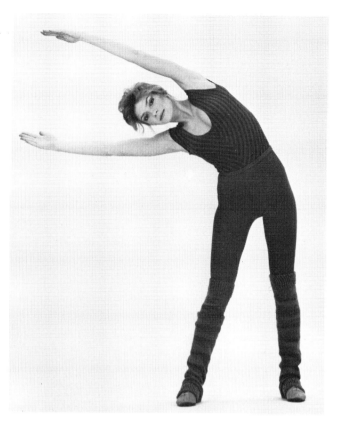

Stretch right.

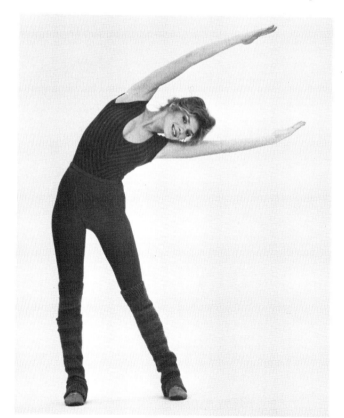

DOUBLE-ARM SIDE STRETCH

Start with arms straight overhead, feet apart, and heels flat on the floor. In an even tilting motion, stretch the arms and torso to the right. Repeat the movement.

Stretch left.

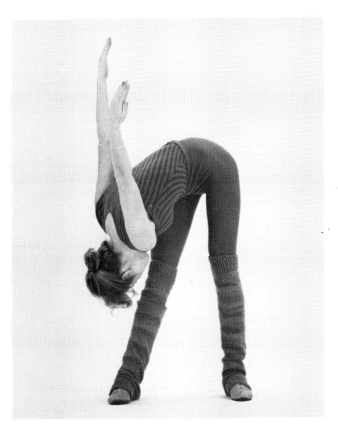

Swing forward to the right leg.

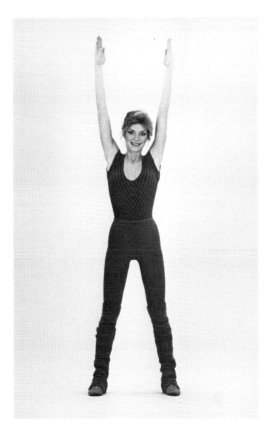

Swing up.

SWING STRETCH

With arms overhead and feet apart, swing forward to the right leg, raising the arms back and up. Swing up, stretching with the arms overhead. Swing forward to the left, raising the arms back and up. Swing up to the original position.

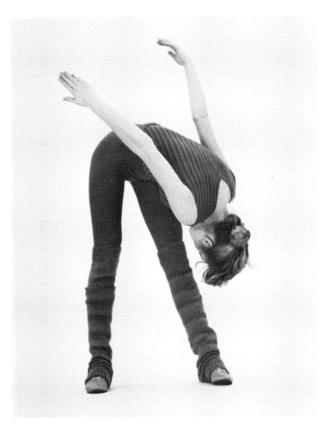

Swing forward to the left leg.

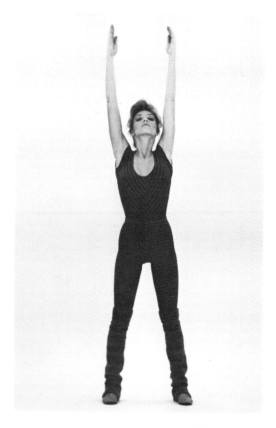

Stretch up.

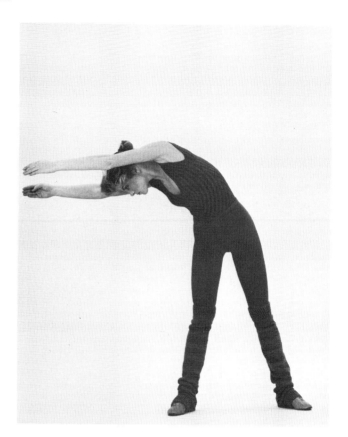

Stretch right.

SWEEP AROUND

Start with arms overhead and feet apart.
Keeping the arms and legs straight, stretch to
the right side and circle down to the floor.
Return, coming up the left side. Alternate
sweeps, stretching right and stretching left.

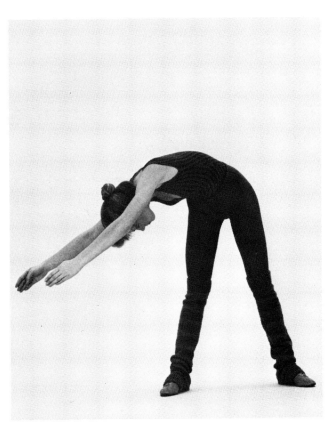

Circle down.

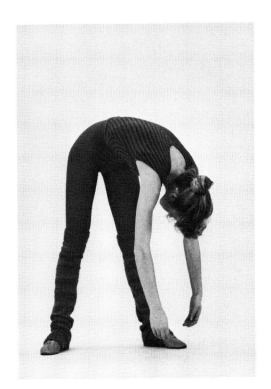

Sweep the floor.

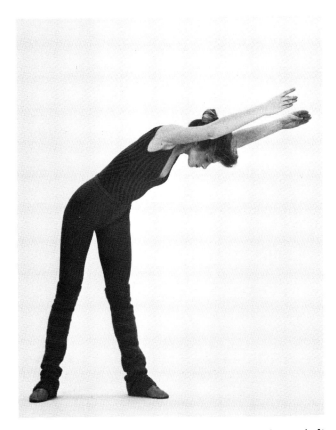

Stretch up left.

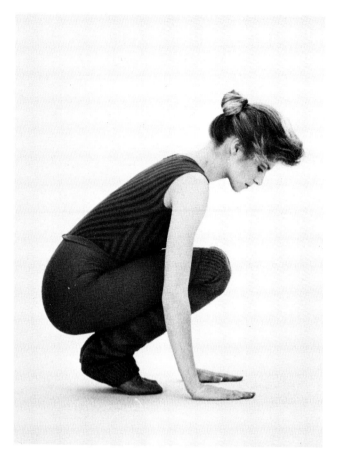

Starting position.

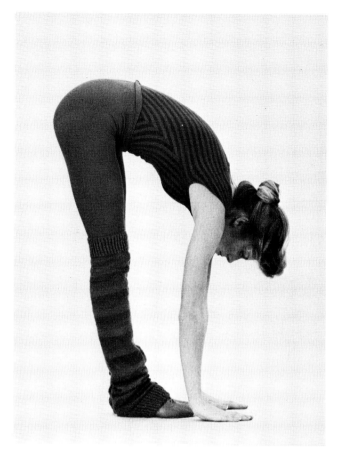

Legs straight.

BEND AND STRETCH

Start in a squatting position with knees bent and relaxed, allowing the heels to come up, palms on the floor. Stretch the legs straight, keeping palms (or fingertips) on the floor. Return to the original relaxed position. Then stand straight up, arms overhead.

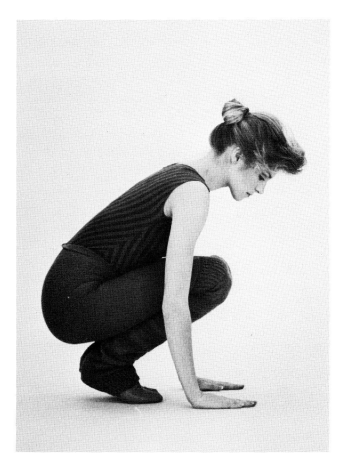

Relax down.

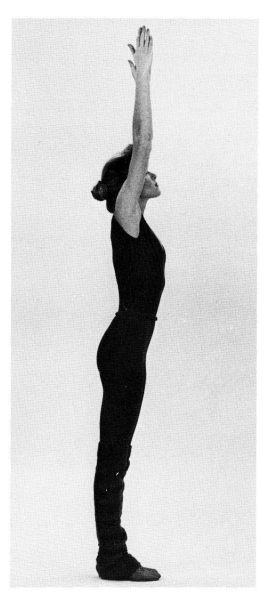

Stand straight up.

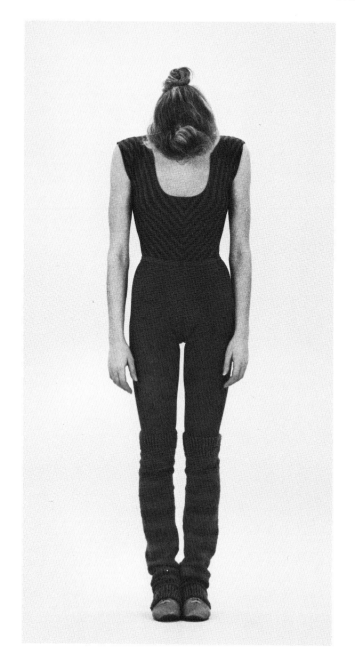

Relax forward.

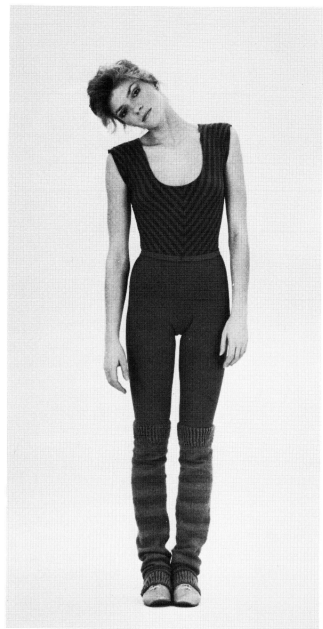

Roll right.

HEAD ROLL

With feet together and arms relaxed at the sides, relax the head forward. Roll the head to the right, relax back, and roll to the left. Repeat the sequence in reverse.

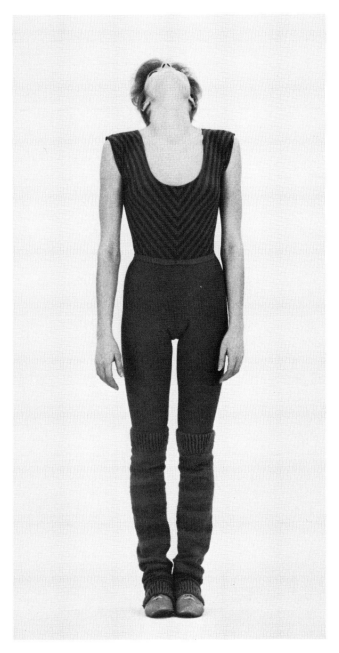

Relax back.

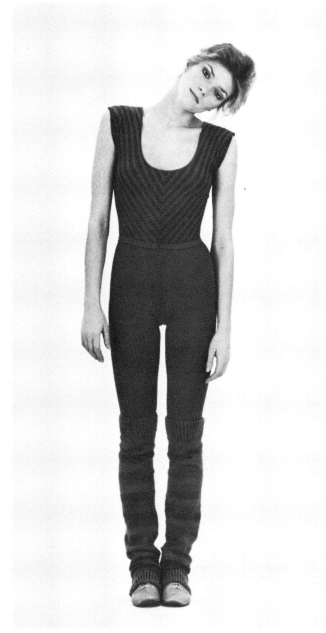

Roll left.

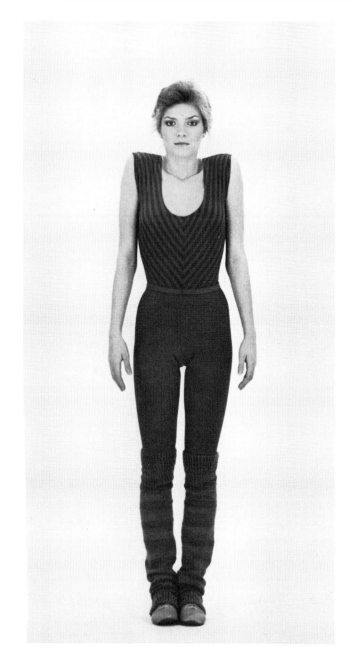

Lift the shoulders.

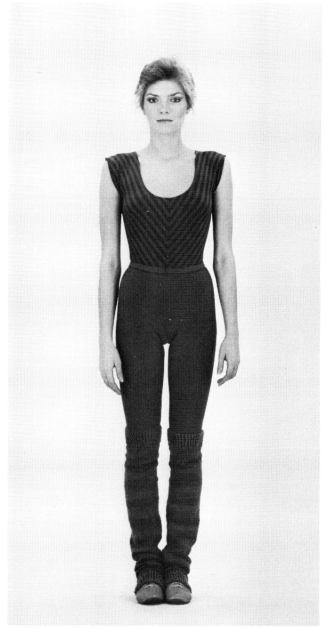

Relax.

SHOULDER SHRUG

With feet together and arms relaxed at the sides, lift up with both shoulders and relax. Lift the right shoulder and relax. Lift the left shoulder and relax.

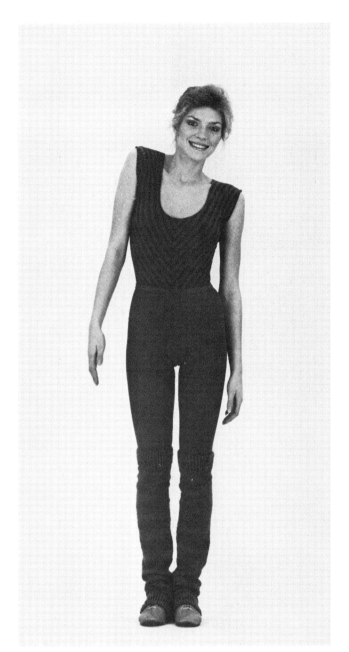

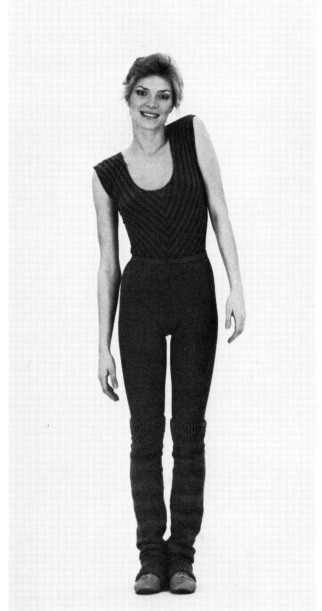

Lift the right shoulder and relax.   *Lift the left shoulder and relax.*

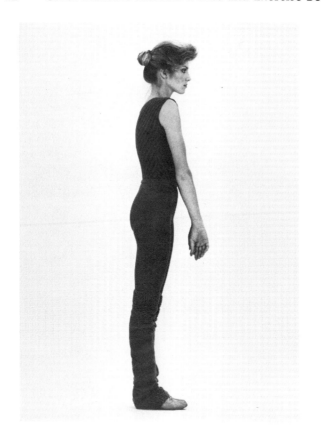

Shoulders forward.

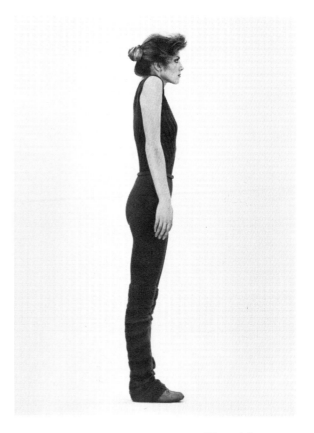

Shoulders up.

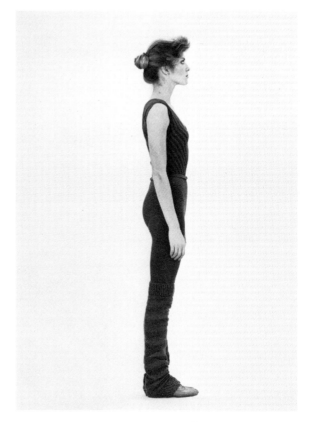

Shoulders back.

SHOULDER ROLL

With feet together and arms relaxed at the sides, roll the shoulders forward, up, and back.

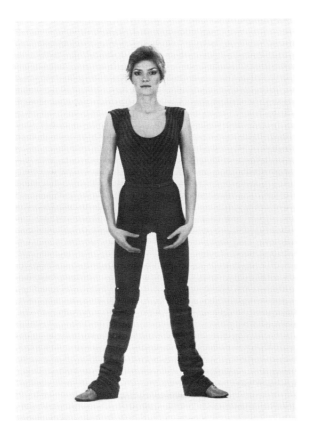

Second position.

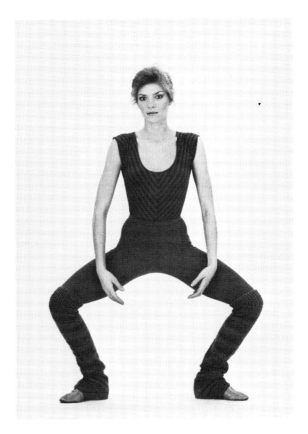

Bend the knees.

PLIÉ

Start with feet apart and turned out in the second position, arms relaxed in front of the body. Slowly come down, bending the knees directly over the toes, keeping the back straight (do not roll the feet inward) and the heels flat on the floor. Straighten up to the original position.

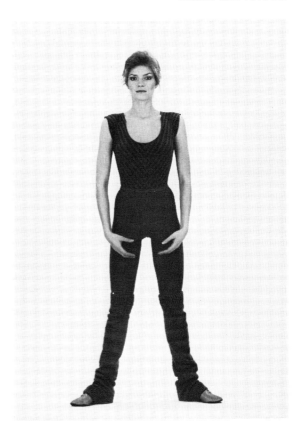

Return to the original position.

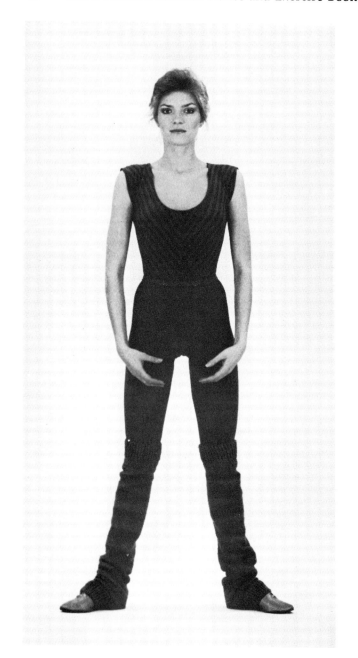

Second position.

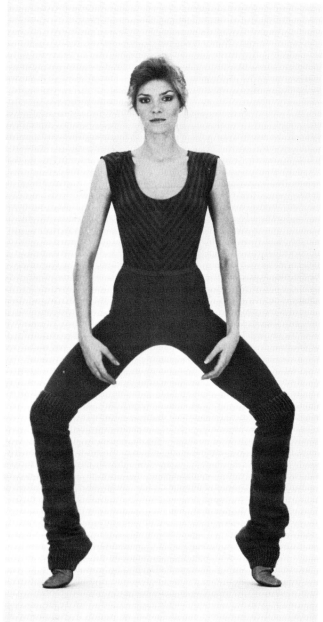

Plié, lifting the heels.

FEET FLEX

Start with feet apart and turned out in the second position, arms relaxed in front of the body. Lift the heels up as you plié. Straighter the legs, keeping the feet flexed. Return to the original position.

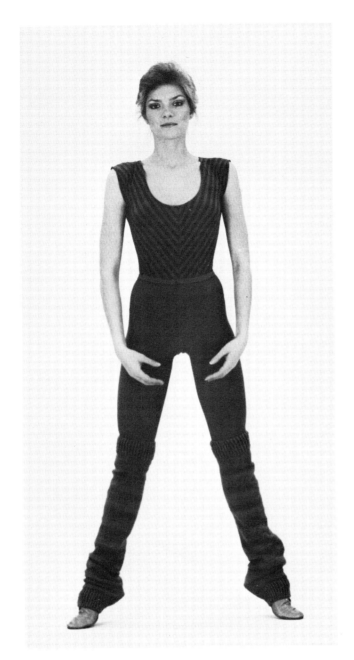

Straighten the legs.

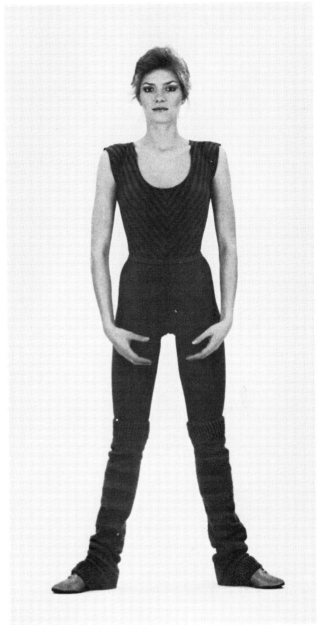

Return to the original position.

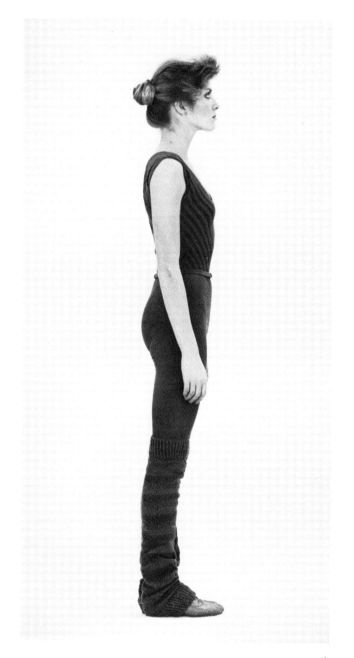

Original position.

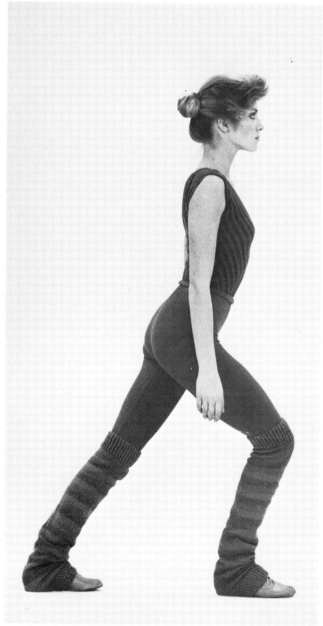

Lunge right.

FORWARD LUNGE

Start with feet together and arms down at the sides. Lunge forward with the right leg, bringing the weight forward and stretching the back leg. The heels should be flat on the floor. Return to the original position and alternate, lunging forward on the left leg.

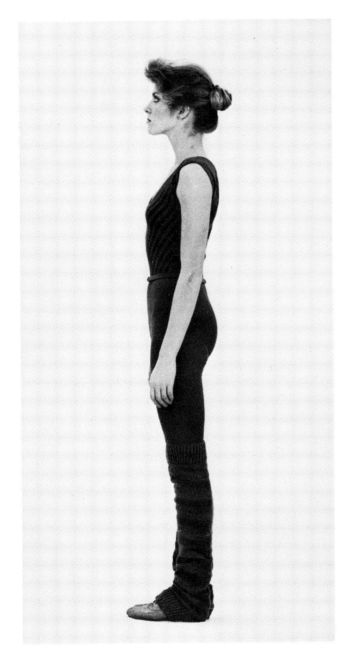

Straighten.

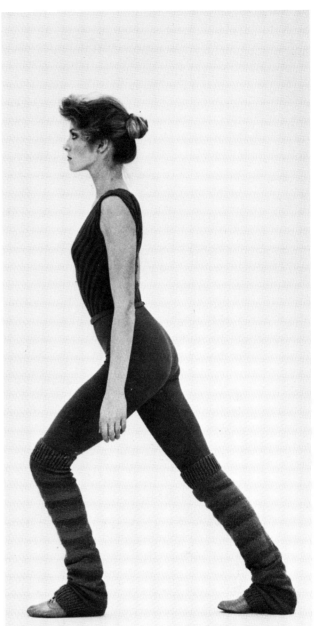

Lunge left.

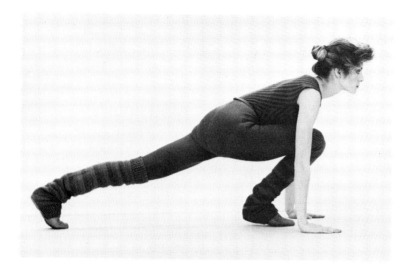

Lunge right.

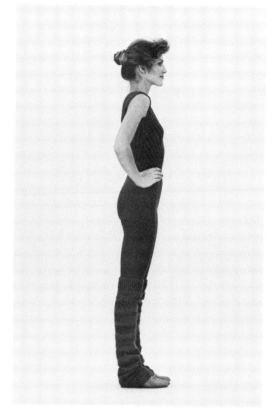

Stand up.

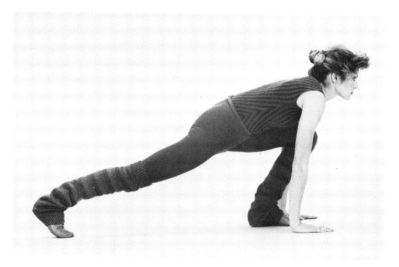

Lunge left.

FORWARD LUNGE TO FLOOR

Lunge forward to the floor on the right leg, with the left leg back and stretched. Stand up, hands on hips, then lunge forward to the floor on the left leg, with the right leg stretched back. Stand up.

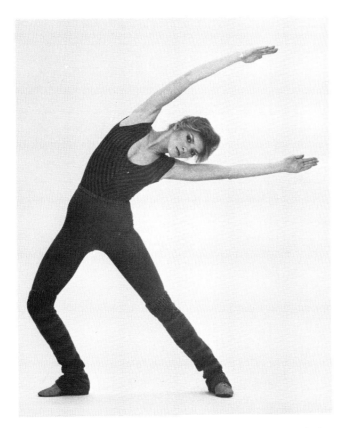

Lunge right.

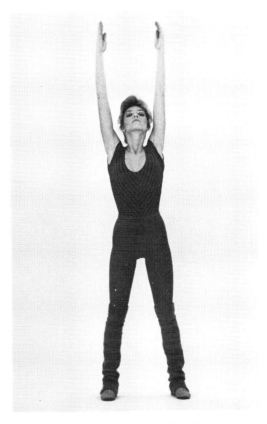

Straighten up.

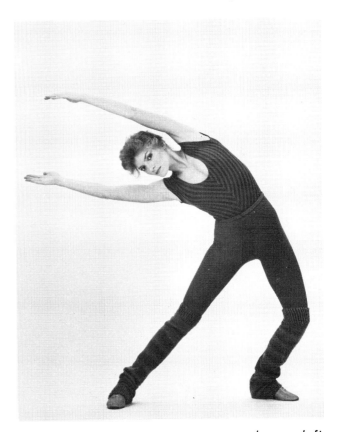

LUNGE

Lunge to the right by bending the right leg and stretching both arms to the left over the straight left leg. Straighten to the center and lunge to the left, bending the left leg and stretching the arms to the right.

Lunge left.

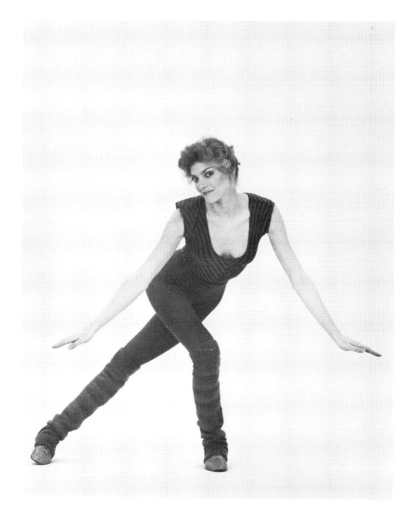

Lunge right, cross left.

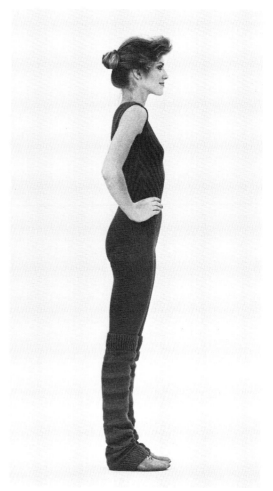

Stand up.

CROSS LUNGE

Lunge forward on the right leg, crossing the left leg in back. The arms should be out to the sides for balance. Stand up, placing the hands on the hips. Repeat the movement, lunging on the left leg and crossing the right leg in back. Stand up.

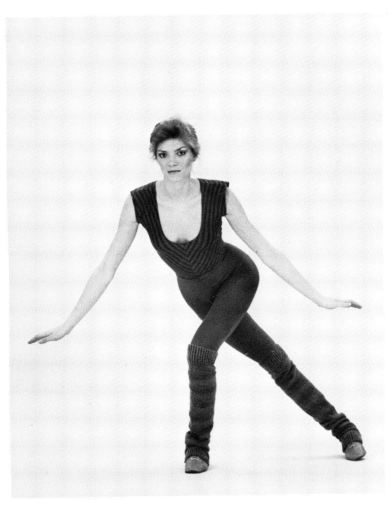

Lunge left, cross right.

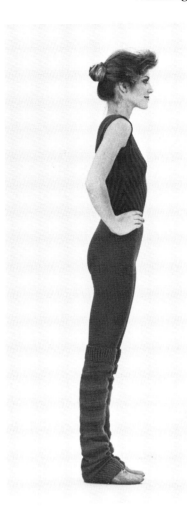

Stand up.

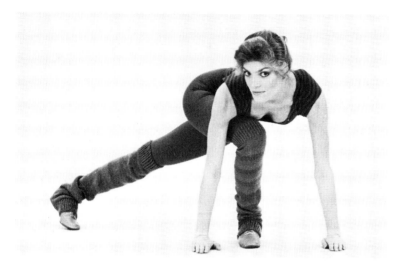

Deep cross, lunge right.

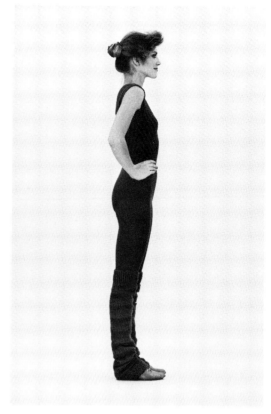

Stand up.

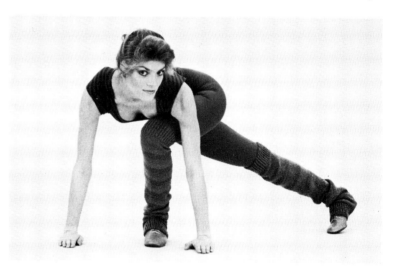

Deep cross, lunge left.

CROSS LUNGE TO FLOOR

Lunge deeply to the floor on the right leg, crossing the left leg in back. The back heel should be up, the weight forward, and palms flat on the floor. Stand up. Repeat the deep lunge to the other side, crossing the right leg in back of the left leg.

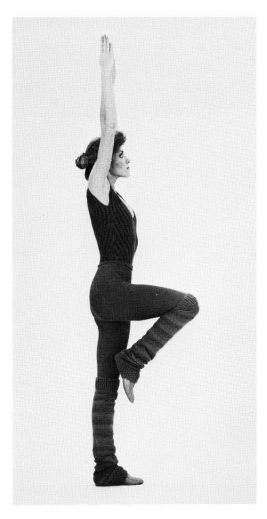

Lift the right leg.

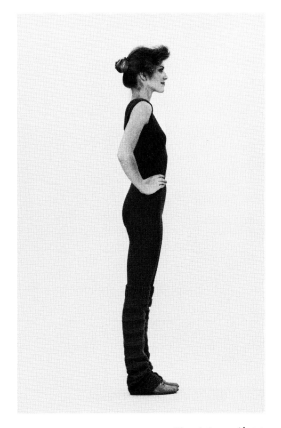

Feet together.

FORWARD BOB

With arms straight overhead, lift the right leg up. Bring the feet together and place the hands on the hips. Bob forward at the waist. Reverse, lifting the leg up, and bob forward.

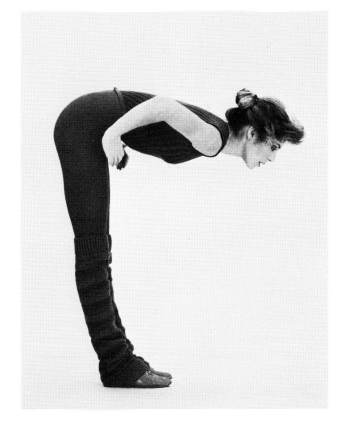

Bob.

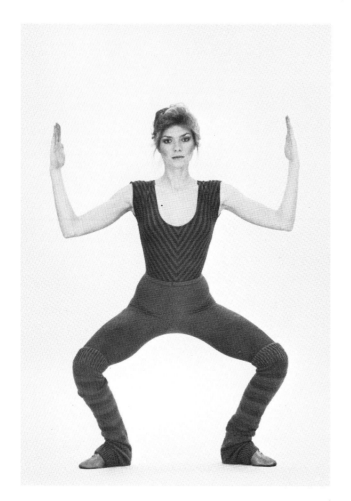

Plié.

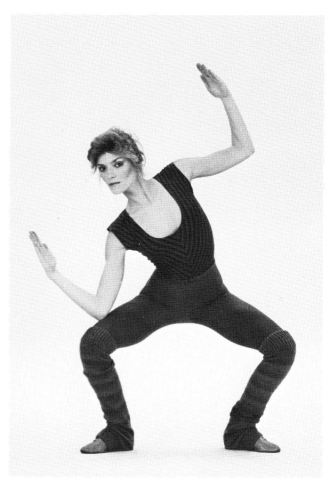

Touch the right knee.

TOUCH PLIÉ

Start in the second position with feet turned out; plié, bending the knees over the toes. Bend to the side, touching the right elbow to the right knee. Then touch the elbows to both knees. Stretch up with arms overhead. Repeat the sequence, touching the left elbow to the left knee.
Good for the upper thighs.

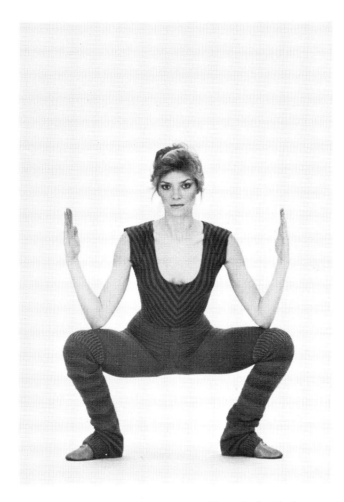

Touch both knees.

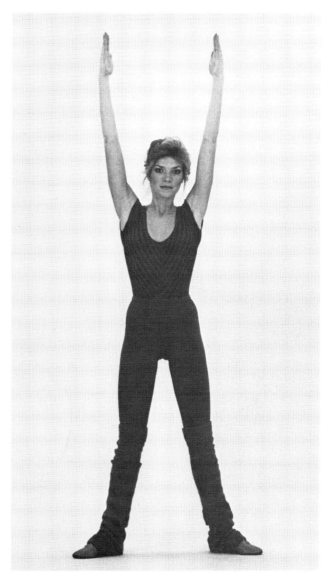

Stretch up.

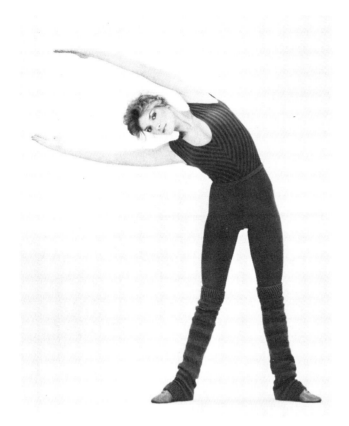

Stretch right.

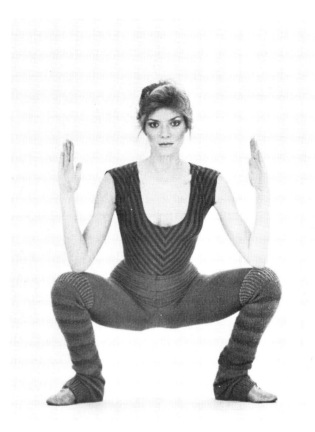

Deep plié, touching elbows.

SIDE STRETCH PLIÉ

With feet turned out in the second position and arms overhead, bend and stretch to the right. Deep plié, touching the elbows to the knees. Then stretch to the left and deep plié. *Good for the upper thighs.*

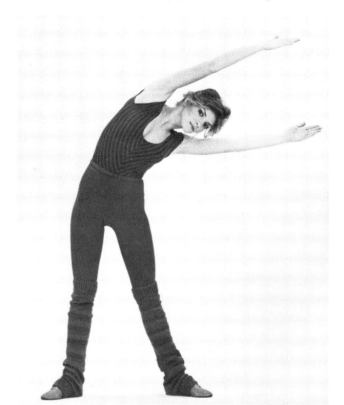

Stretch left.

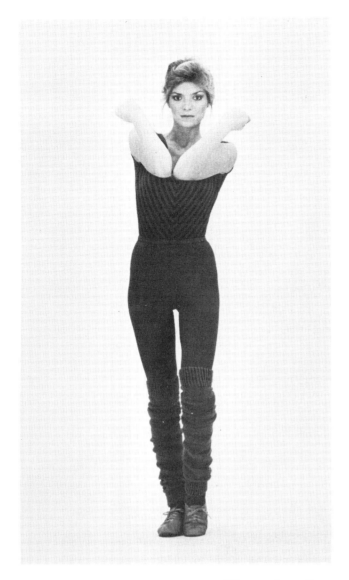

Elbows together.

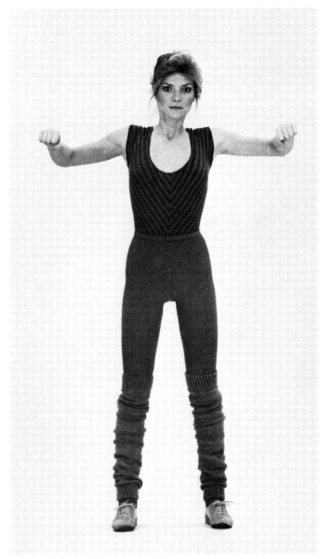

Swing back.

ELBOW TOUCH

With feet apart, touch the elbows in front,
keeping the fists out. Swing the elbows back.
Be sure to keep the shoulders and arms level.
Good for the upper arms and back.

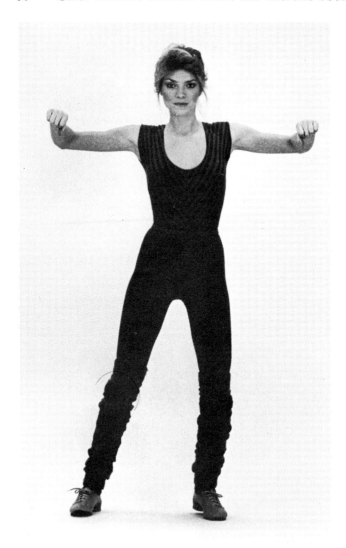

Step out, elbows back.

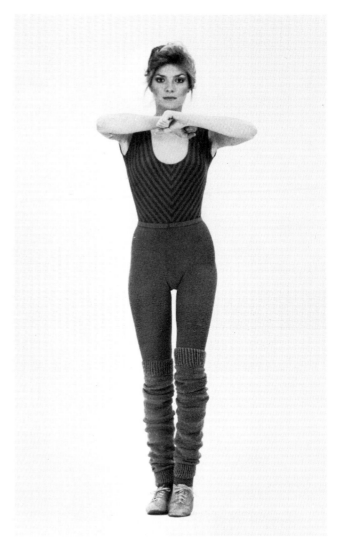

Feet together, arms in.

ELBOW SWING AND SIDE STEP

Step to the right with the right leg and swing the elbows back. Step to bring the feet together and swing the arms in. Step out again, swinging the elbows back. Touch with the left foot. Repeat the movement, stepping out with the left foot and touching with the right foot.
Good for the waistline and upper back.

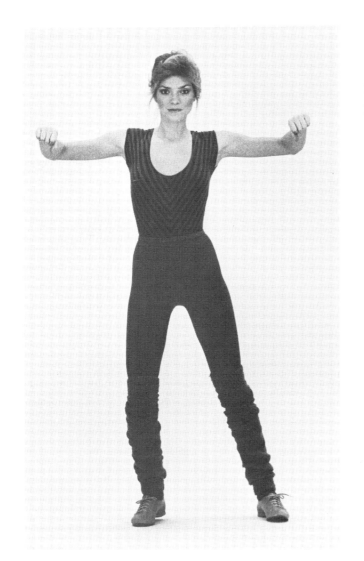

Step out, elbows back.

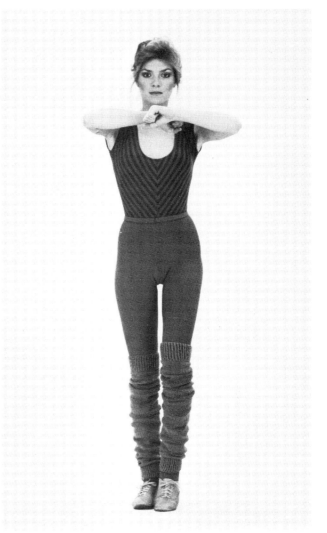

Feet together, arms in.

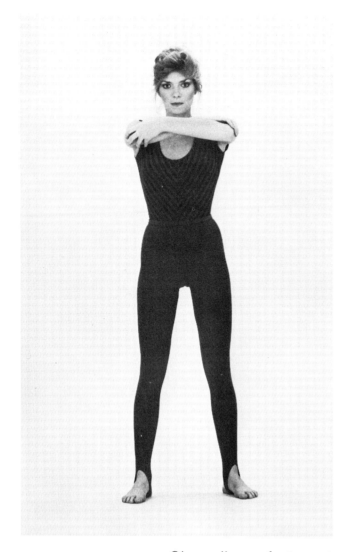

Clasp elbows, feet apart.

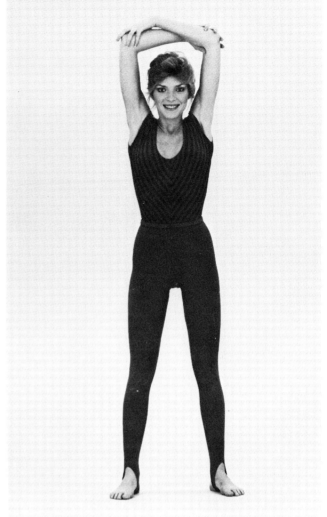

Lift arms overhead.

ELBOW LIFT AND SWING

Start with feet apart, hands clasping elbows,
raised to shoulder level. Lift the arms
overhead and then lower them to the waist.
Lift the arms and swing from side to side,
keeping the arms at shoulder level.
Good for the waistline and upper back.

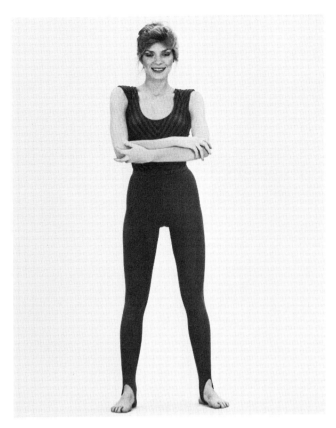

Lower arms to waist.

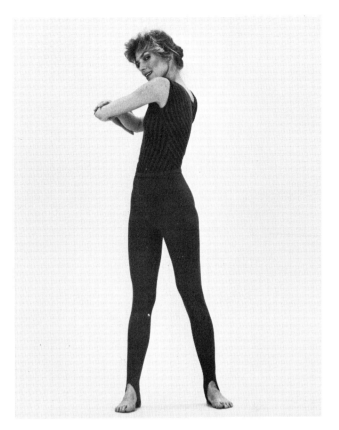

Swing to the right.

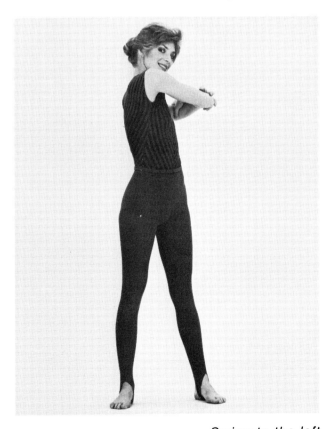

Swing to the left.

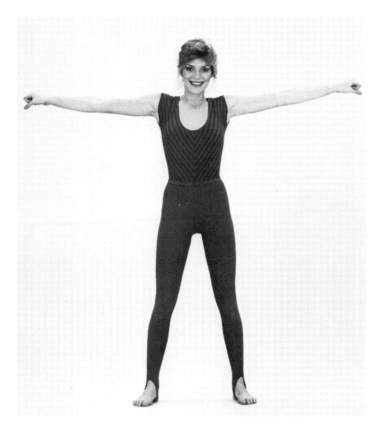

Arms out.

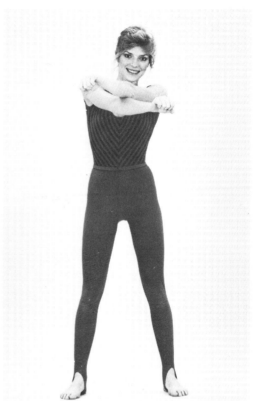

Cross in front.

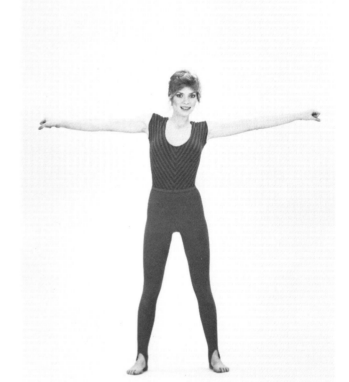

Swing back.

ARM SWING

With feet apart, extend the arms straight out to the sides at shoulder level. Make fists. Cross the arms in front and swing back. *Good for the waistline and upper back.*

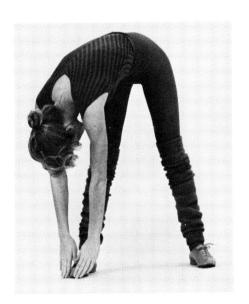

Touch right.

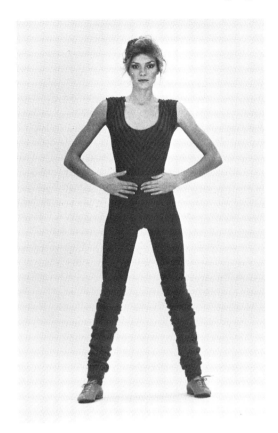

Tap center.

TOE TOUCH

With feet apart, bend at the waist and touch both hands to the right toes. Stand up and tap the center of your waist. Bend and touch the left toes.
This is a good hip isolation exercise.

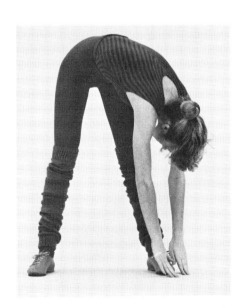

Touch left.

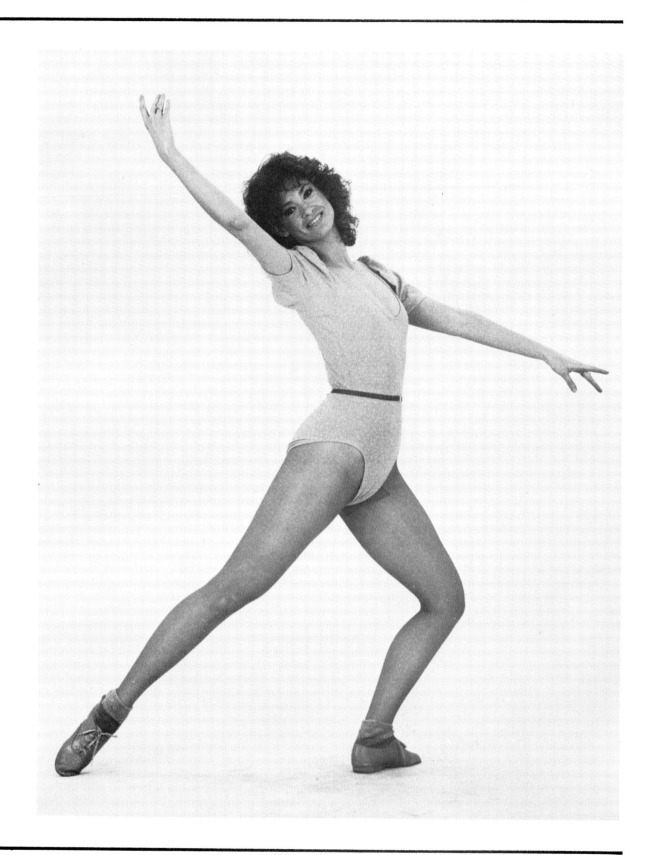

6

Dance Steps and Exercises

As soon as you have warmed up and stretched for at least 10 minutes, go directly into the dance routines using the suggested steps and exercises that follow. Do not take time to cool off.

During the routines, try to maintain a steady pace. That way your heart will beat at a regular rate and you will not become easily fatigued as a result of pushing yourself too hard for a short period of time. If you become out of breath or find that you cannot keep in step, simply slow down and perhaps do every other beat. Some of my students drop their arms to their sides and just keep time to the music by stepping lightly from side to side until they've regained their strength. If you prefer a shorter aerobic workout, cut down on the number of routines and go right into the cool-downs. Remember that, with continued activity, your entire body, including the muscles and cardiovascular system, will become stronger and the routines will become easier.

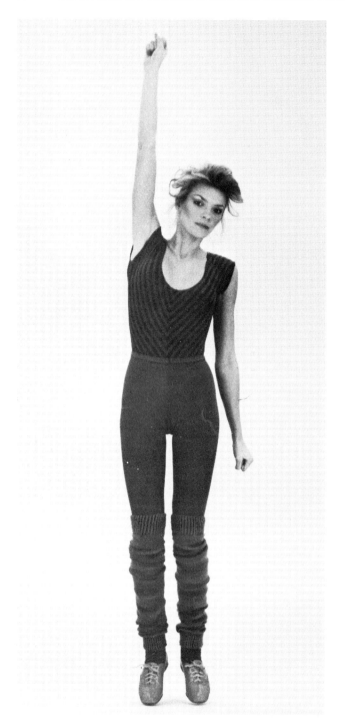

Jump right twice.

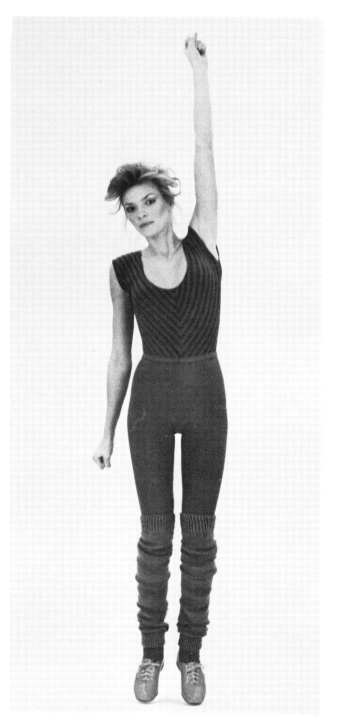

Jump left twice.

POGO

Start with feet together and arms at your sides. Jump twice to the right on both feet and raise the right arm. Repeat the movement to the other side.

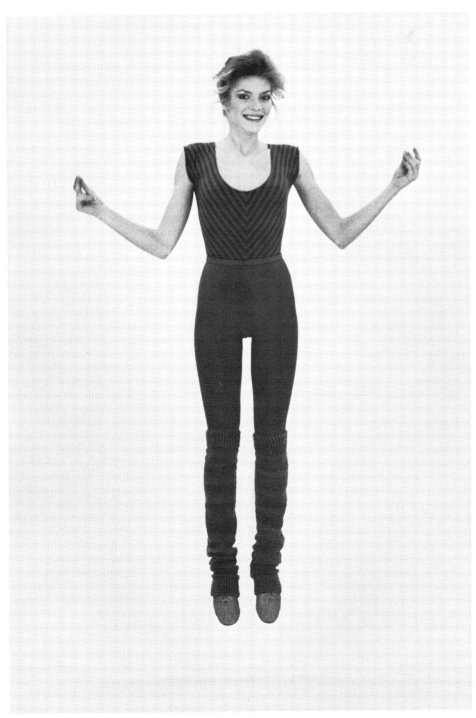

Jump in place, snap fingers.

JUMP IN PLACE

Jump in place while snapping your fingers.

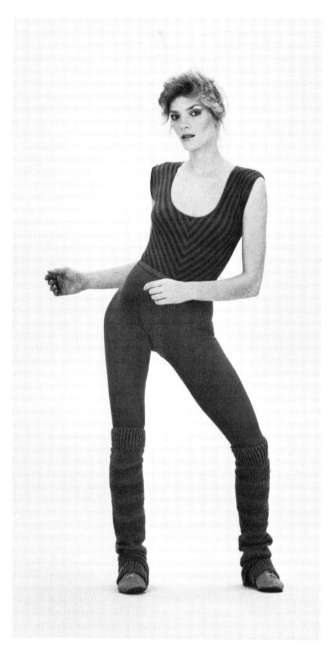

Step right, swing hip.

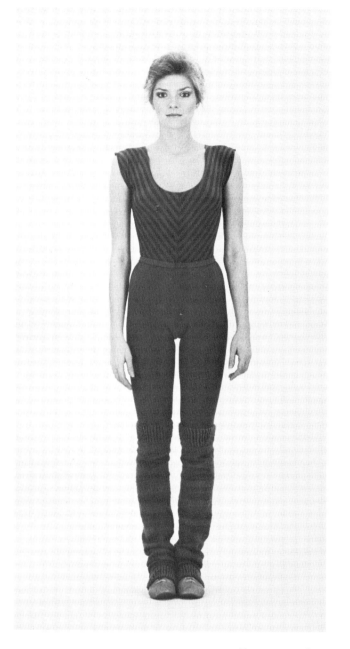

Feet together.

HIP SWING WITH SIDE STEP

Step out with the right foot and swing the right hip and the arms. Step together; step out; touch with the left foot. Repeat with the left foot.

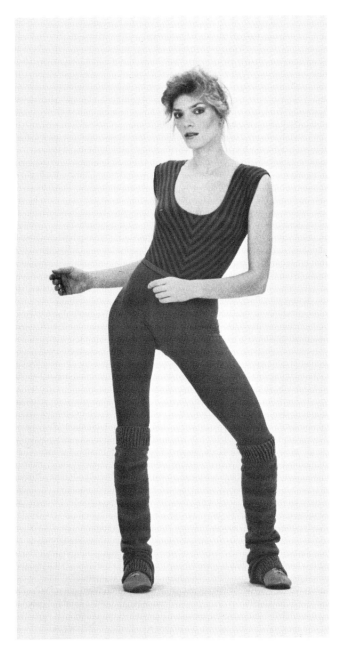

Step right.

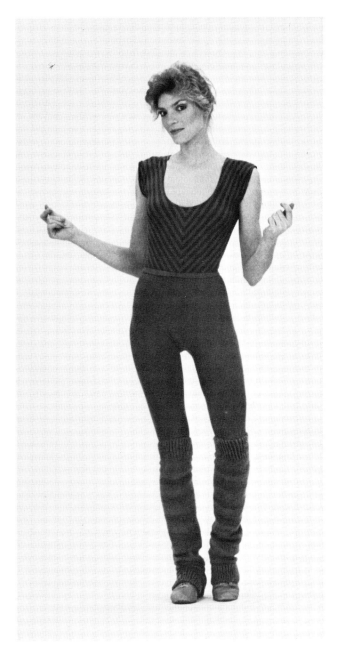

Touch with the left foot.

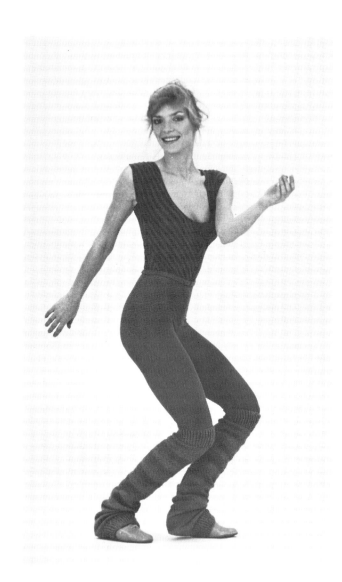

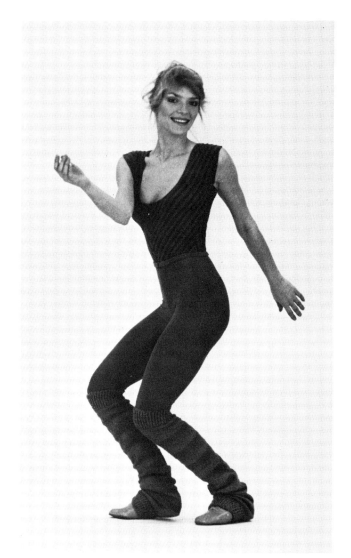

Twist right.

Twist left.

TWIST

With feet apart, twist to the right and twist to the left, moving the hips.

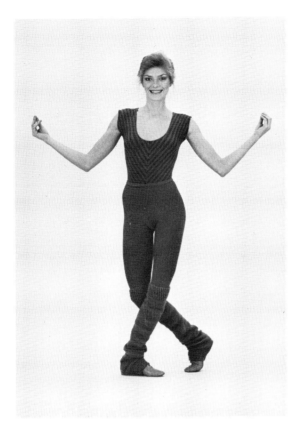

Starting position.

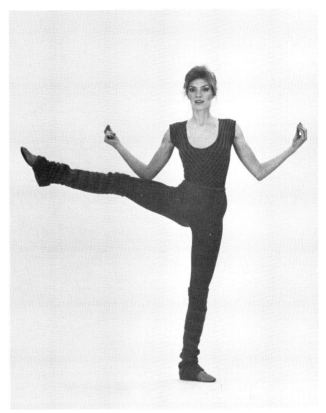

Kick to the side.

SIDE FLICK KICK

With the left foot turned out and carrying the weight, position the right leg in back, knee bent and foot flexed. Kick the right leg out to the side and bring it back. Repeat with the other leg.

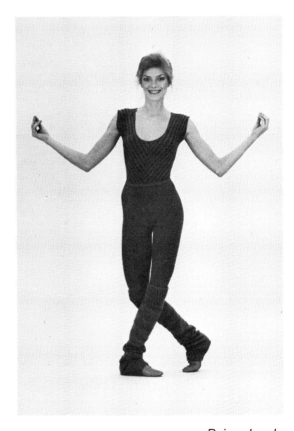

Bring back.

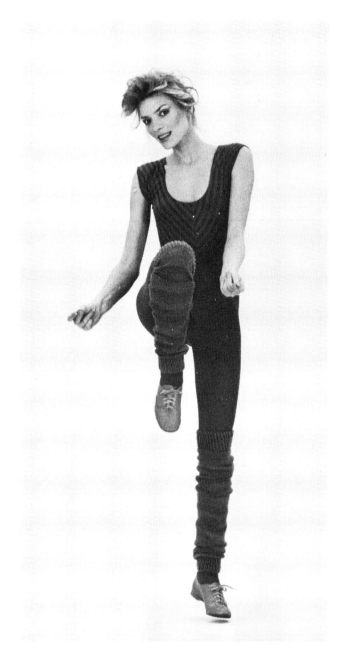

Lift the right knee.

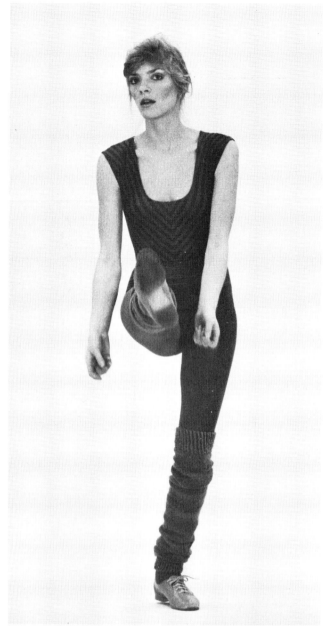

Kick the right leg.

HOP FLICK KICK

Hop as you lift the right knee up. Kick the
right leg out. Hop to the left leg and lift the
knee.
This exercise is good for the legs and raises the heart rate.

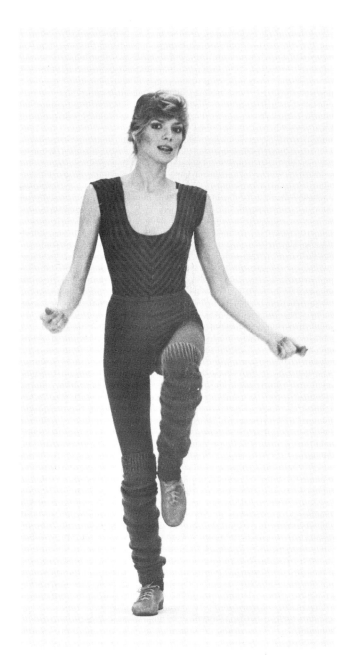

Hop and lift the left knee.

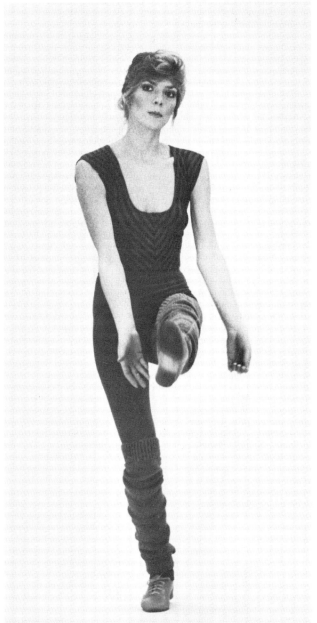

Kick the left leg.

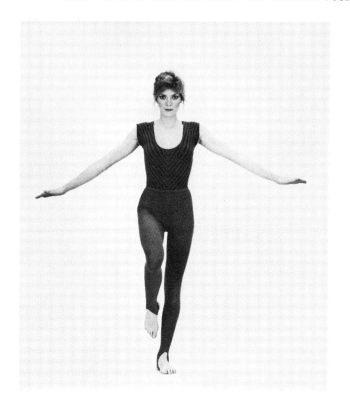

Hop.

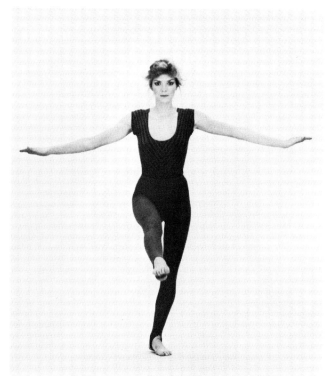

Hop, kick to the front.

FLICK KICK FRONT AND SIDE

With arms out at the sides, hop onto your left foot. Hop and kick forward with the right leg. Hop and kick to the side with the right leg. Repeat, alternating legs.

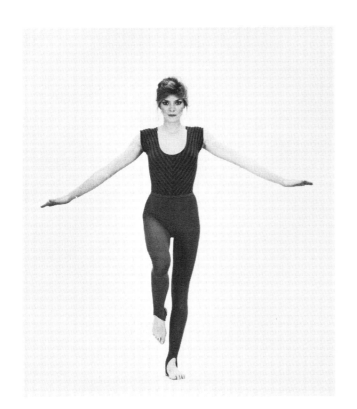

Hop.

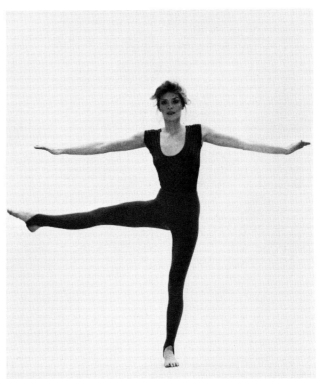

Hop, kick to the side.

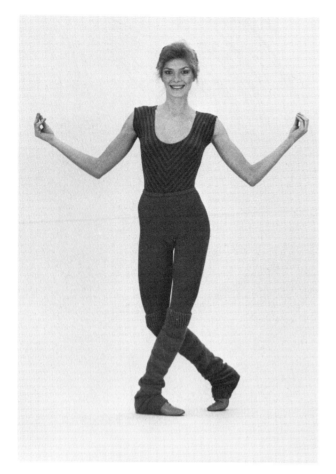

Right leg back.

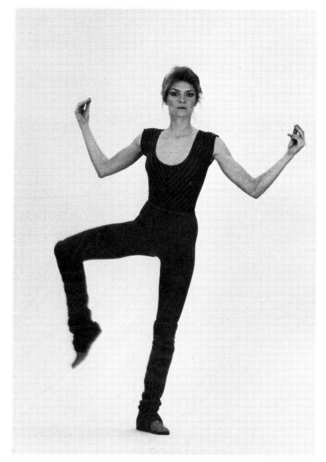

Flex the right knee.

SIDE KICK AND CROSS OVER

With left foot turned out and carrying the weight, position the right leg in back, knee bent and foot flexed. Flex the right knee to the side at waist level. Kick the right leg high to the side. Cross the right leg in front of the left. Repeat the movement with the other leg.

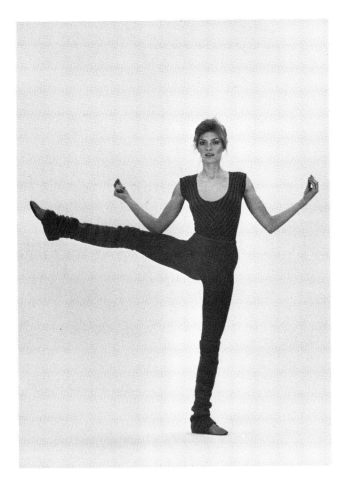

Kick high.

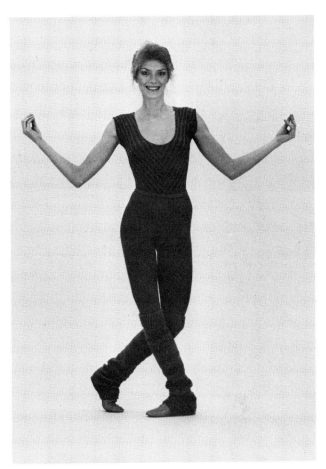

Cross over the left leg.

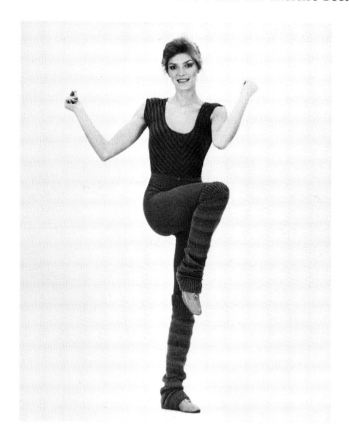

Touch the right knee to the left elbow.

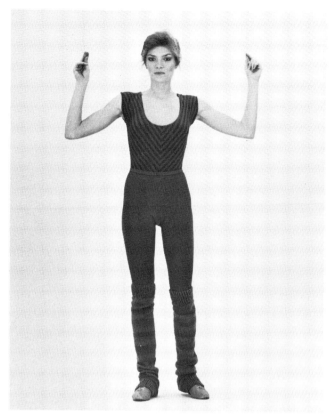

Return to the original position.

KNEE LIFT I

Begin by lifting the right knee to the left elbow. Drop the leg to the original standing position. Alternate, lifting the left knee to the right elbow. Be sure to lift the knee up to the elbow without bending at the waist, keeping back straight.

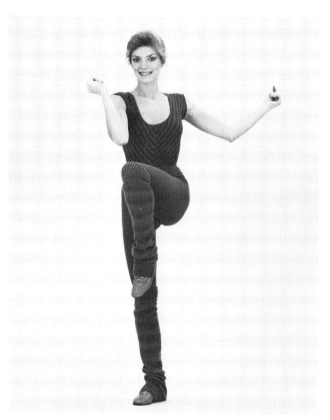

Touch the left knee to the right elbow.

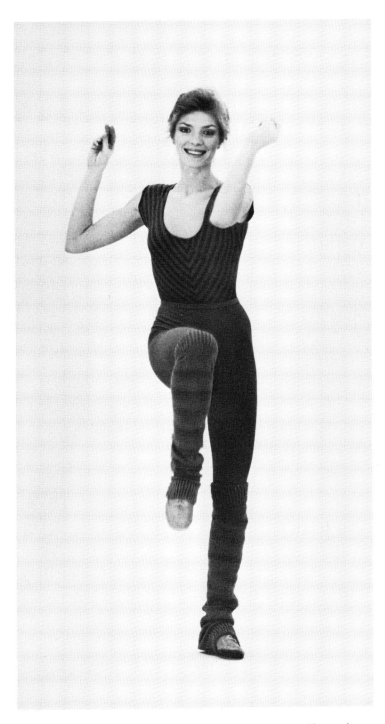

Knee hop.

KNEE HOP

Hop as you touch the right knee to the left
elbow and the left knee to the right elbow.

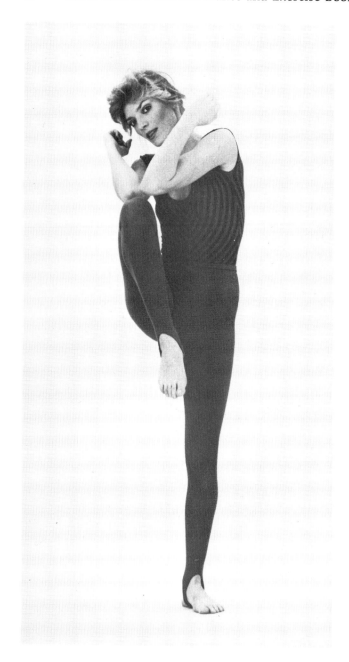

Touch the right knee to both elbows.

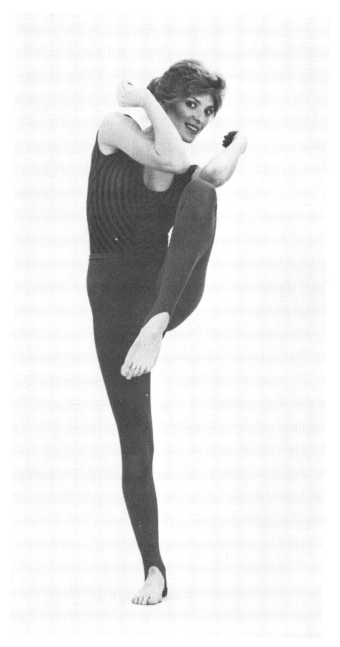

Touch the left knee to both elbows.

KNEE LIFT II

Begin by lifting the right knee to both elbows
at the same time. Repeat the movement,
lifting the left knee.

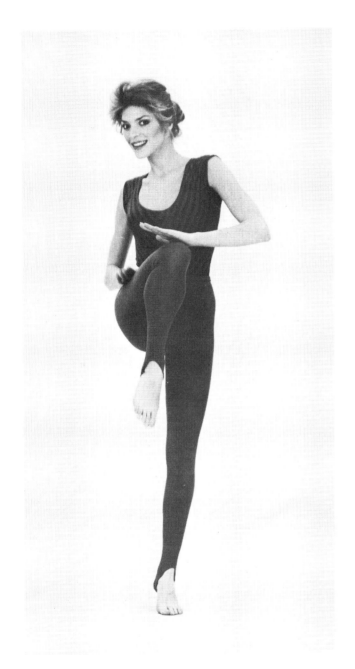

Hop right, slapping the right knee.   *Hop left, slapping the left knee.*

KNEE SLAP

Hop as you lift the right knee and slap it with both hands. Repeat the step, slapping the left knee.

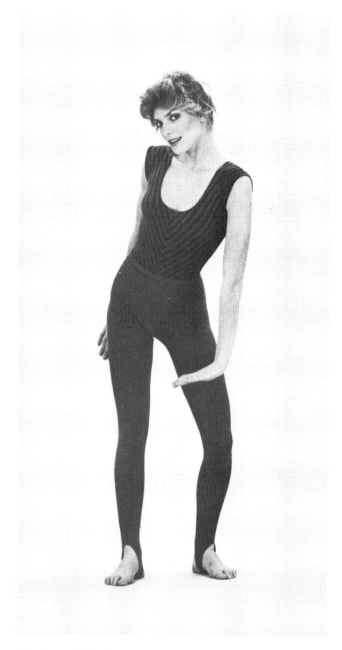

Shake right, two counts.

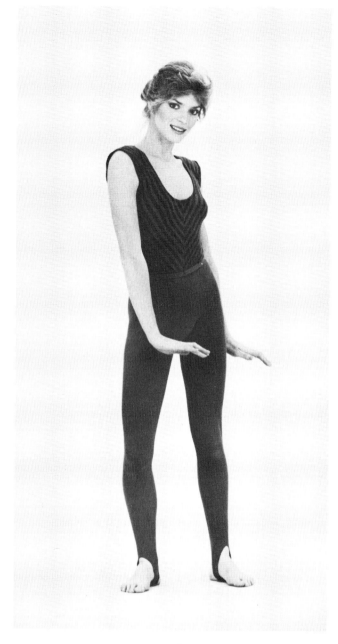

Shake left, two counts.

KNEE BOUNCE AND HIP SLAP

With knees slightly bent, shake the hips to
the right and push down, with hands flexed,
for two counts. Then push down and shake
the hips to the other side for two counts. Lift
one arm up and shake for two counts. Lift
both arms up and shake for two counts.

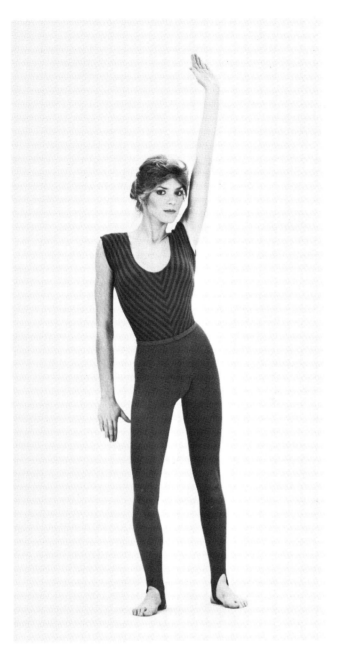

Arm up, two counts.

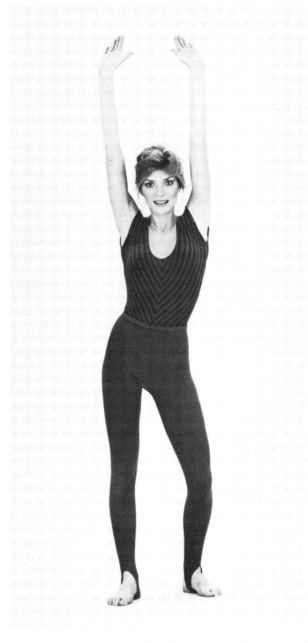

Both arms up, two counts.

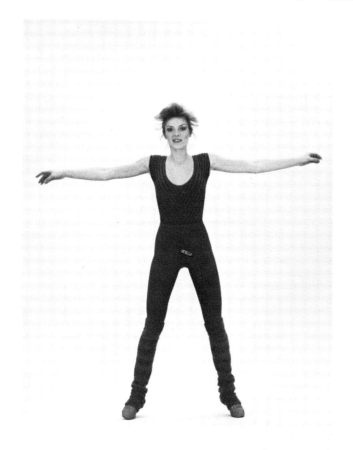

Jump in place.

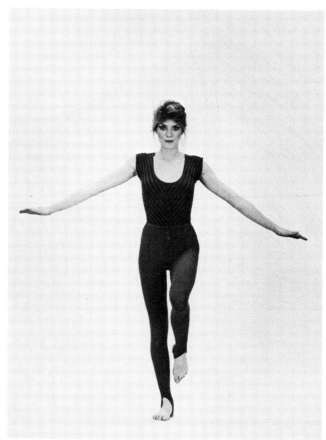

Jump and hop, right foot.

HOPSCOTCH

With feet apart and arms out to the side, hop
in place. Jump onto the right foot and hop.
Hop in place; jump onto the left foot and
hop.

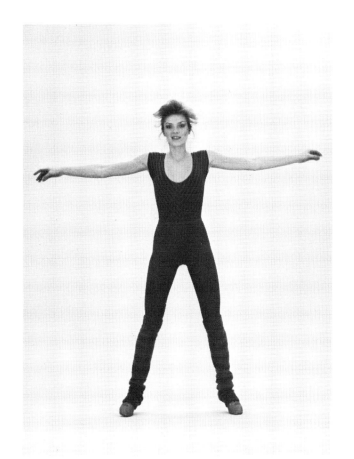

Hop.

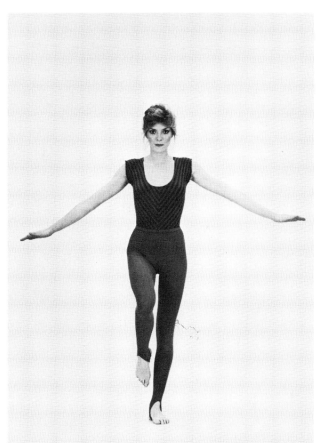

Jump and hop, left foot.

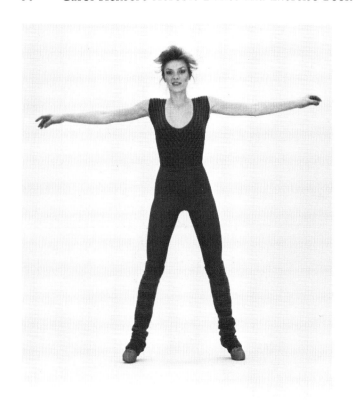

Jump in place.

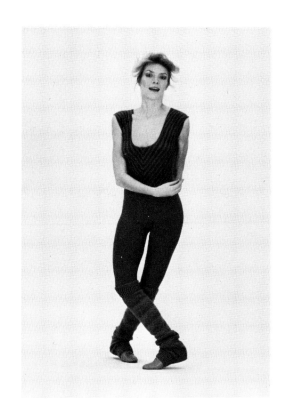

Jump and cross.

JUMP CROSS

With feet apart and arms out to the side, jump in place. Jump and cross feet. Jump out; jump and cross alternating feet.

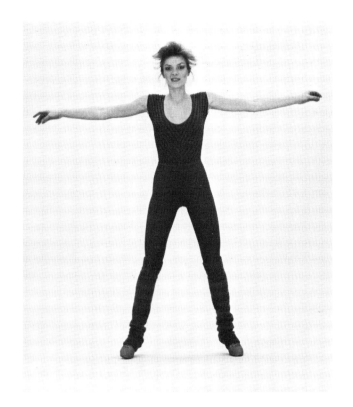

Jump out.

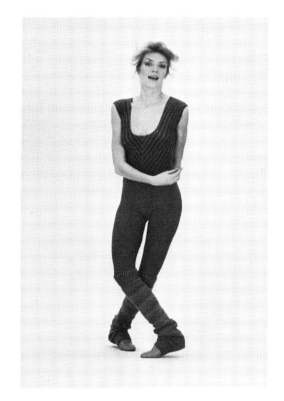

Jump and cross.

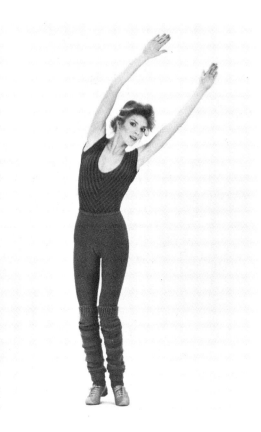

Jump right, stretch left.

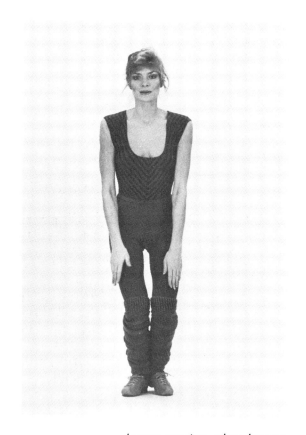

Jump center, slap knees.

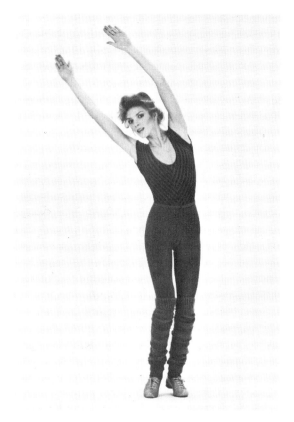

JUMP STRETCH

With feet together and arms overhead, jump to the right and stretch to the left. Jump to the center and slap the knees. Jump to the left and stretch to the right.

Jump left, stretch right.

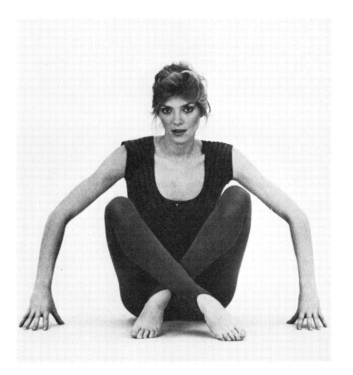

Cross legs, sitting.

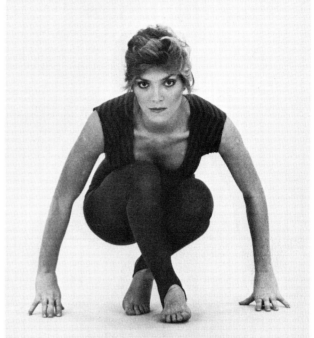

Push forward.

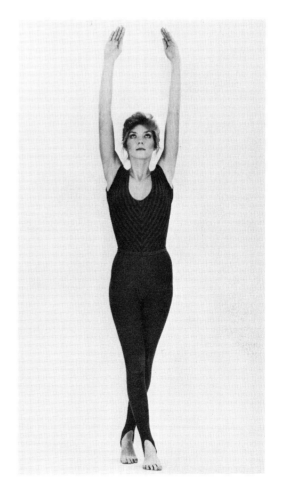

STAND

Sitting on the floor with legs crossed and knees lifted, push forward, using the hands for balance. Lift to a standing position.

Stand up.

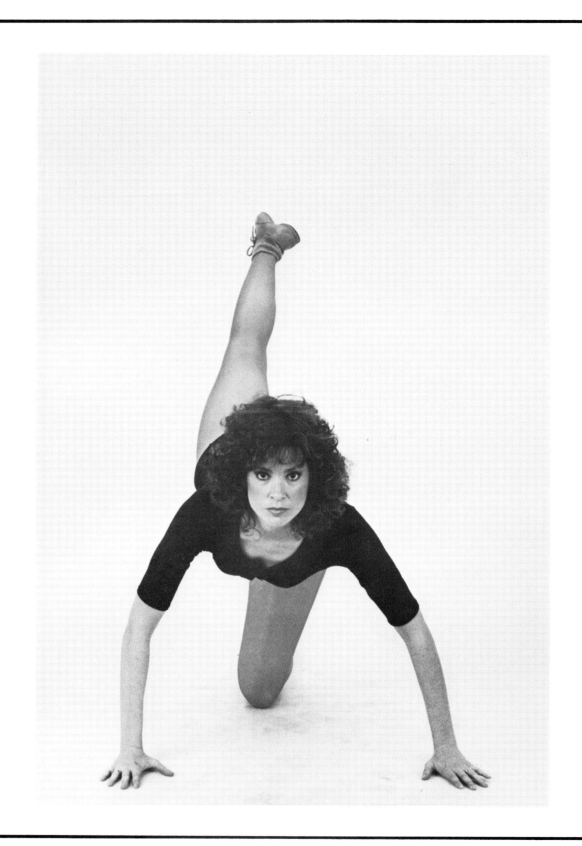

7

Cool-Downs

Not only do cool-downs keep the muscles stretched out until they have returned to the normal body temperature; they also prevent the blood from pooling in the muscles and veins. Perform the cool-downs slowly with gentle dance steps and walking patterns that allow your heart rate to return gradually to its normal level. Remember to keep moving. Walk around the room for 60 seconds. Take your pulse. If your pulse has not dropped to 120 beats or less, continue walking another 60 seconds or until your heart rate comes down.

FLOOR EXERCISES

After your pulse has dropped to 120 beats or below and leveled off, start the floor exercises. These cool-down and stretch-flexibility movements are designed for relaxation and a gradual tapering off from an active workout. Take at least 10–12 minutes to complete them.

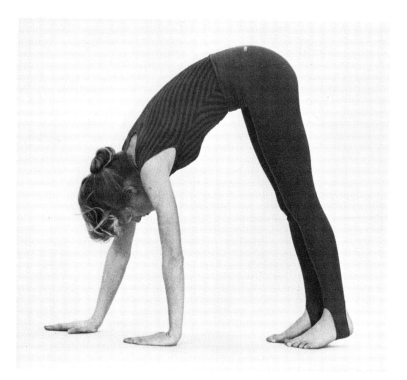

Walk backward.

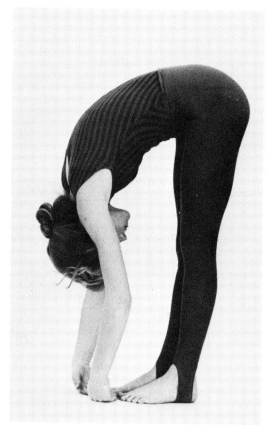

Relax forward.

BACK AND LEG STRETCH

Bend at the waist and place the palms on the floor four feet in front of the toes. The feet should be together. Walk backward, keeping the legs straight. Relax forward. Lift up and flatten the back, arms stretched out in front. Stretch up.

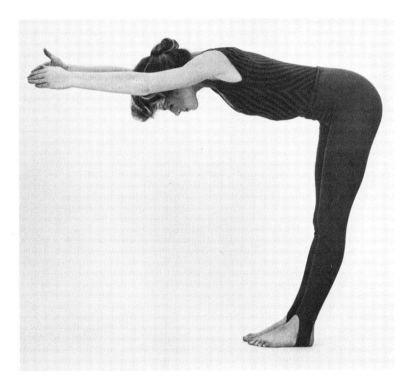

Flatten back.

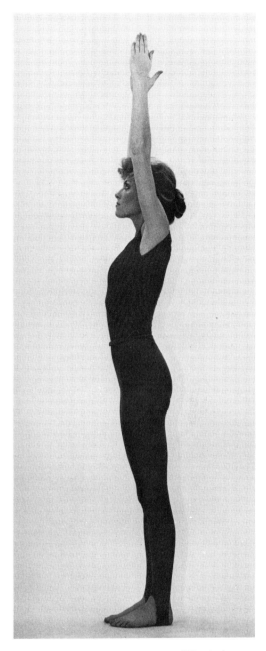

Stretch up.

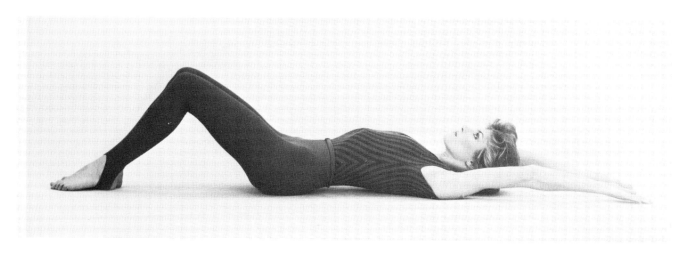

Starting position.

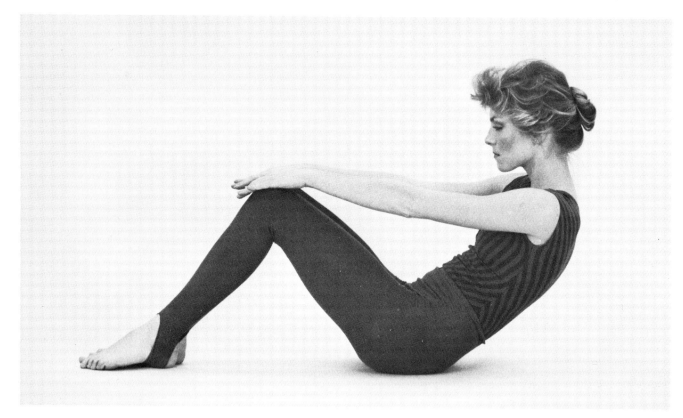

Touch the knees.

RHYTHMIC SIT-UP

Lie flat on the floor, arms overhead, knees
bent and raised off the floor. Lift the torso up
and touch the knees. Touch the toes. Lie
back down to a starting position.

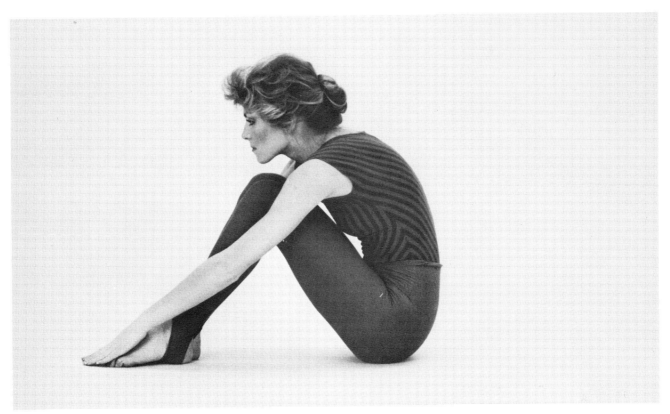

Touch the toes.

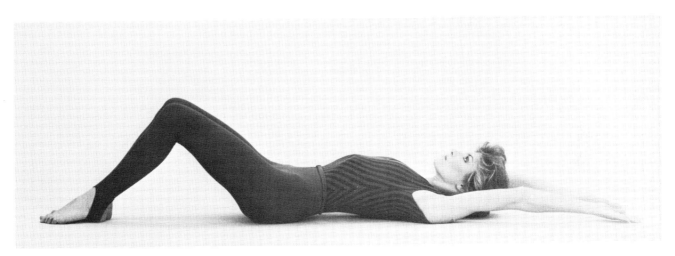

Original position.

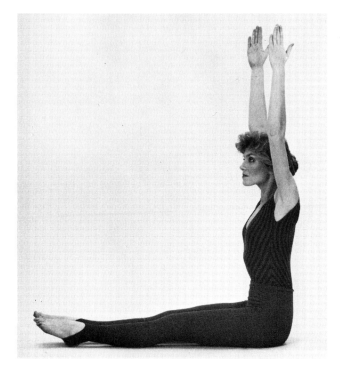

Starting position.

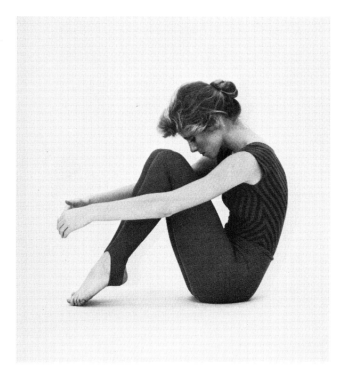

Tuck in.

SWING SIT-UP

Sitting on floor with arms overhead and legs extended straight, pull the legs in toward the chest and lower the arms. Straighten legs and extend arms slowly out to the side and above head, until flat on the floor. Raise upper body to tuck position; extend legs and straighten arms over head to finish.

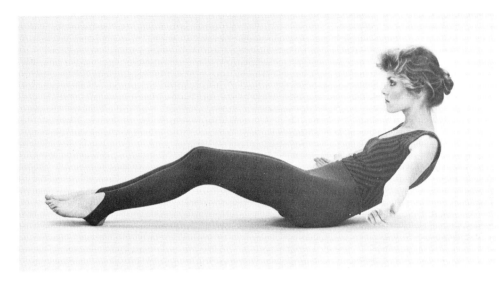

Extend down until flat.

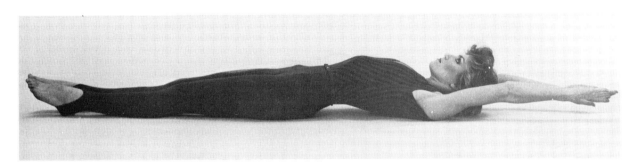

Lie flat.

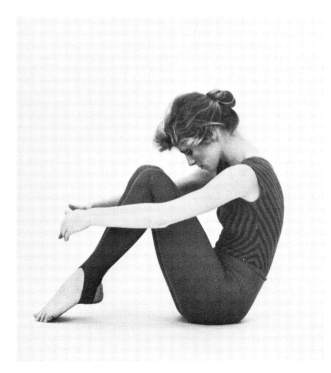

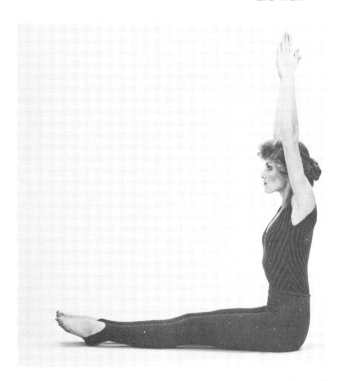

Tuck in.   *Straighten legs and extend arms overhead.*

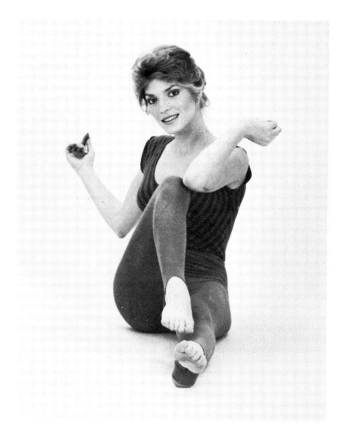

Right knee to left elbow.

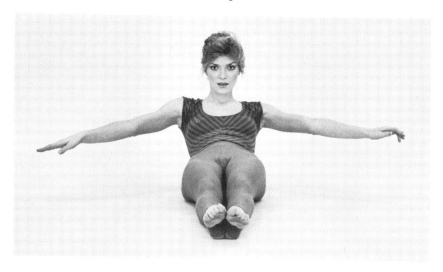

Lie back.

ELBOW TOUCH SIT-UP

Sitting on the floor with legs together in front, lift the right knee and touch it to the left elbow. Lie back, arms out to the side. Lower all the way down to the floor, arms overhead. Repeat the movement, touching the left knee to the right elbow.

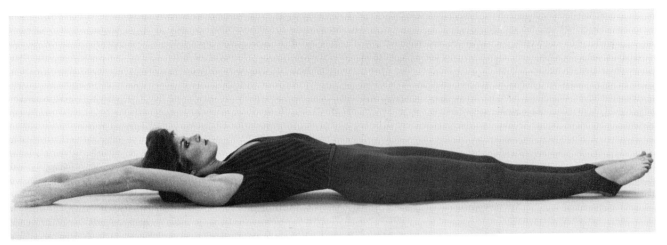

All the way down.

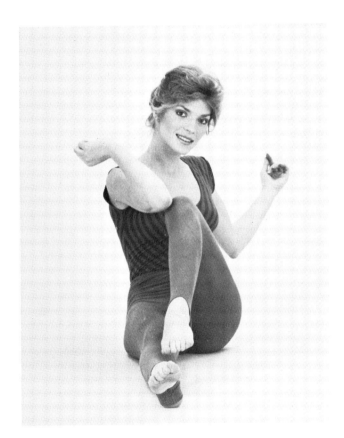

Left knee to right elbow.

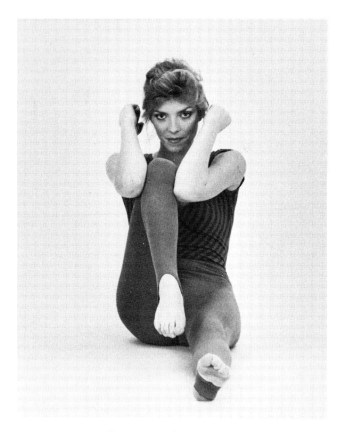

Touch right knee to both elbows.

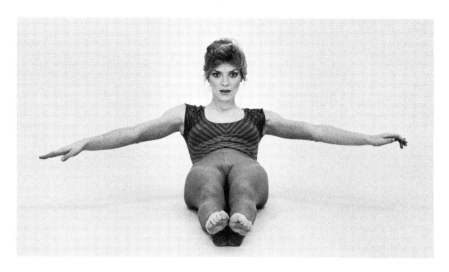

Lie back.

DOUBLE-ELBOW SIT-UP

Sitting on the floor with legs extended in
front, lift the right knee and touch it to both
elbows. Lie back, bringing the arms out to
the side. Lie down all the way to the floor,
arms overhead. Repeat to the opposite knee.

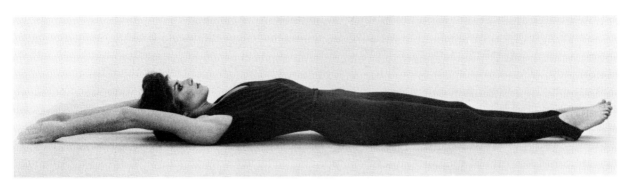

Lower to the floor, arms overhead.

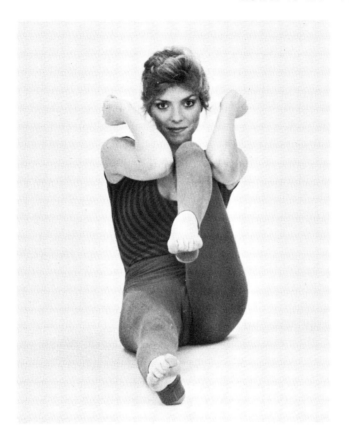

Touch left knee to both elbows.

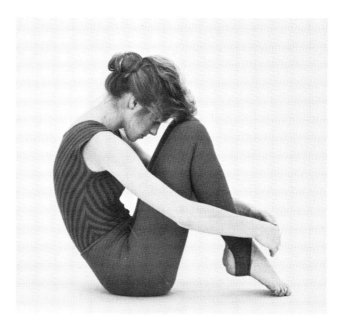

Tuck in.

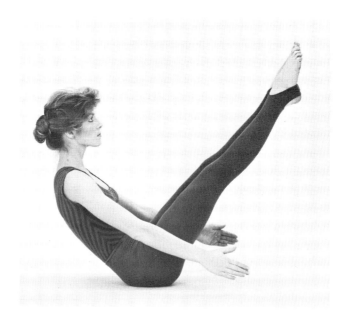

Extend out, legs up.

BALANCING SIT-UP

Sitting on the floor, tuck the knees in to the forehead under the arms. Extend the legs out, 45 degrees off the floor. Tuck in to the original position. Release and lie back, continuing all the way to the floor.

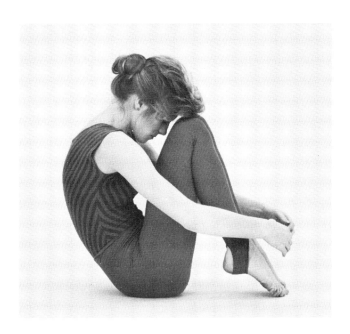

Tuck in.

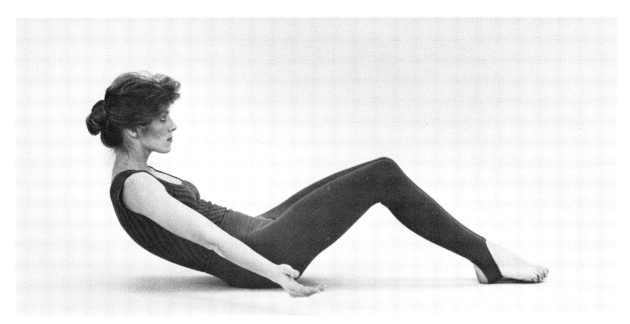

Lie back.

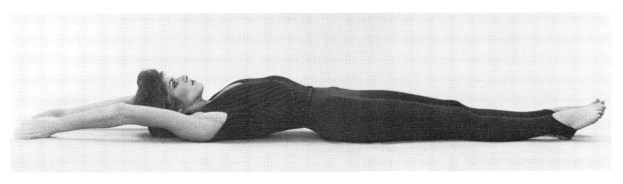

All the way down.

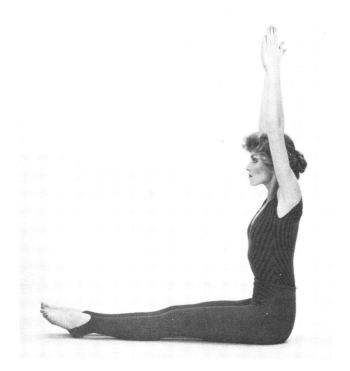

Starting position.

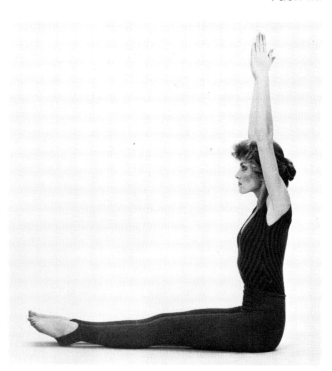

Tuck in.

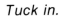

Extend out.

TUCK-IN SIT-UP

With arms overhead and legs together and extended forward, tuck in by bringing the knees in to the chest. Extend out to the original position. Repeat.

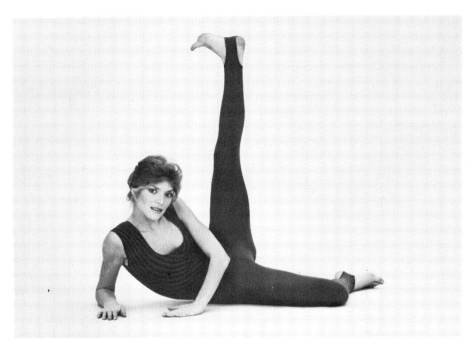

Lift leg, ankle flexed.

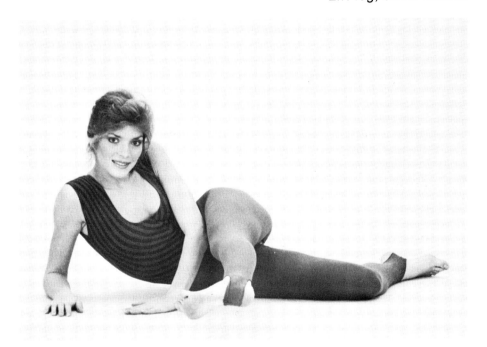

Stretch down and front.

LEG STRETCH I

Lie on your right side. Lean on the right
elbow and keep the torso slightly raised. Use
the left hand for additional support. Raise the
left leg straight up with the ankle flexed.
Bring the leg straight down and forward.
Stretch. Repeat on the other side.

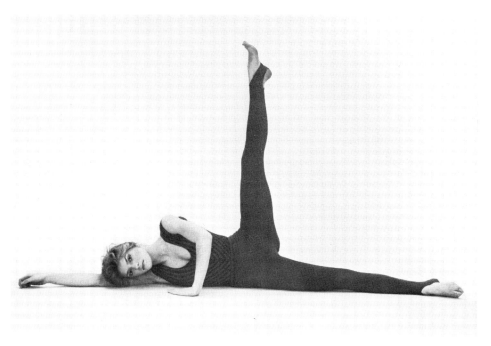

Kick left leg up, stretch straight.

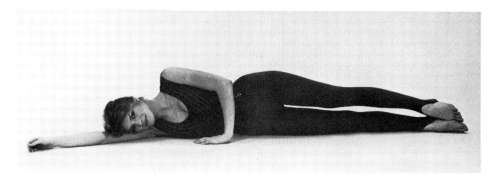

Relax down.

SIDE LEG KICK

Good for hips and upper thighs. Lie on your right side with the right arm extended overhead. Use the left hand for balance. Kick the left leg straight up and relax down. Repeat the movement on the other side.

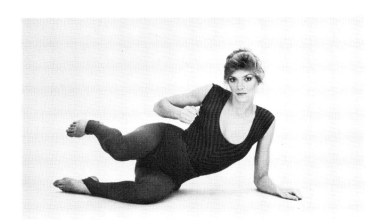

Tuck in.

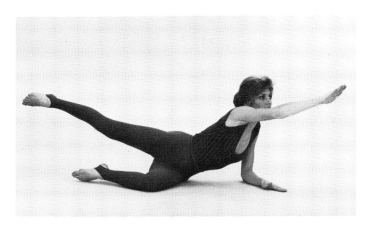

Stretch kick.

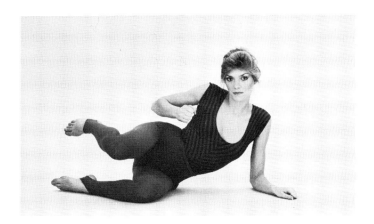

Tuck in.

TUCK STRETCH KICK

Good for back of hips and waist. Lie on your left side. Tuck the legs in. Lean on the left elbow and keep the torso slightly raised. Extend the right arm forward and kick the right leg back, lifting it as high as possible. Tuck back in.

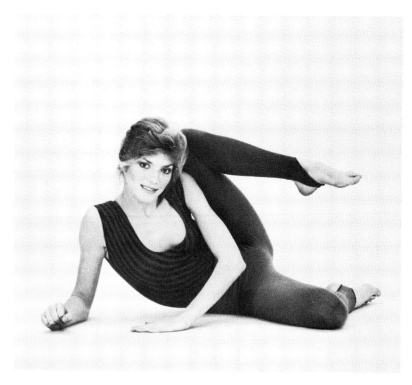

Tuck in.

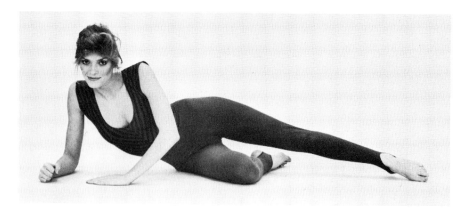

Stretch down.

TUCK SIDE LEG KICK

Good for upper thighs. Lie on your right side.
Lean on the right elbow and keep the torso
slightly raised. Use the left hand for
additional support. Bend the knees and tuck
the feet in. Raise the left leg, bringing the
knee to the shoulder. Extend the leg out and
lower it. Kick the left leg up and stretch.
Lower the extended leg to the floor. Repeat
the sequence on the other side.

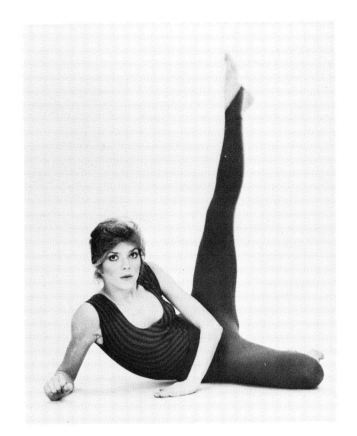

Kick up.

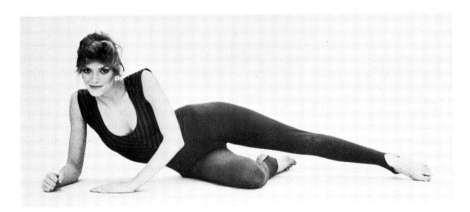

Stretch down.

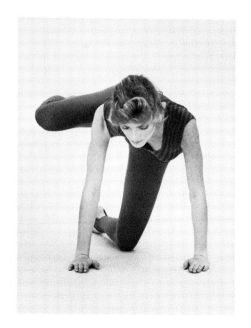

Flex.

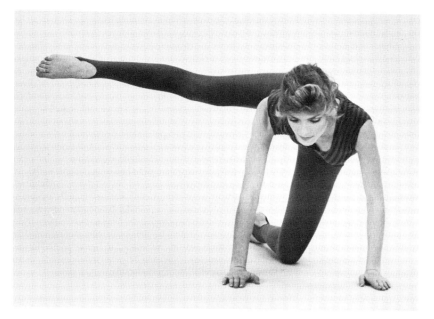

Kick.

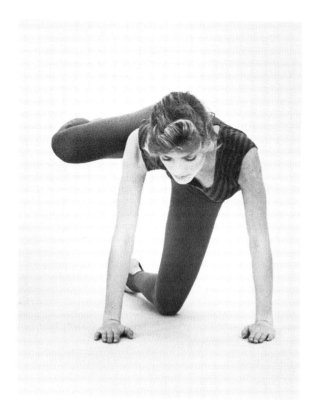

Flex.

SIDE FLEX KICK

Good for hips. Rest on your hands and knees. Lift the flexed right leg out to the side. Kick and extend the leg. Flex back. Repeat the sequence with the other leg.

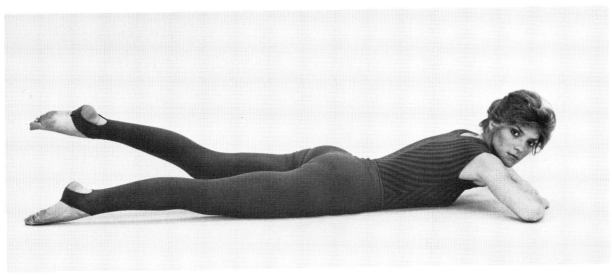

Flutter kick left.

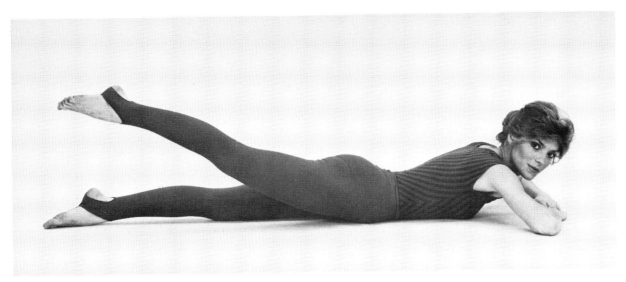

Flutter kick right.

FLUTTER KICK

Lie face down, arms bent. The legs should be together, toes pointed. Grip the buttocks tightly and lift the legs, alternating kicks, bringing the entire legs off the floor. The movement comes from the hip.

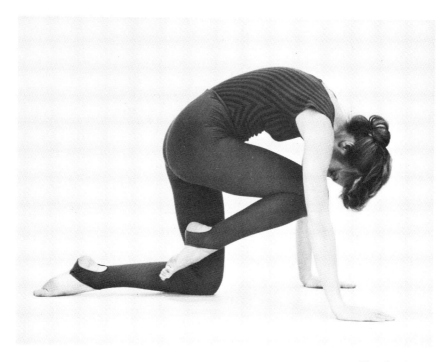

Tuck right.

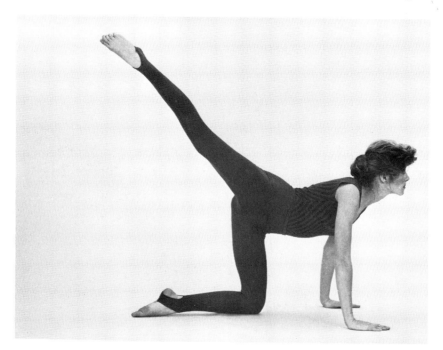

Kick right.

DONKEY KICK

Good for buttocks. Rest on your hands and knees. Lift and tuck in the right knee to the chin. Kick the right leg straight back and stretch up, lifting your head. Repeat the sequence with the other leg.

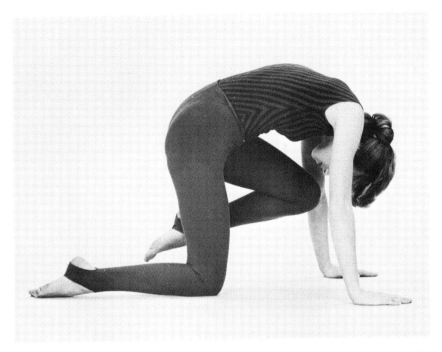

Tuck left.

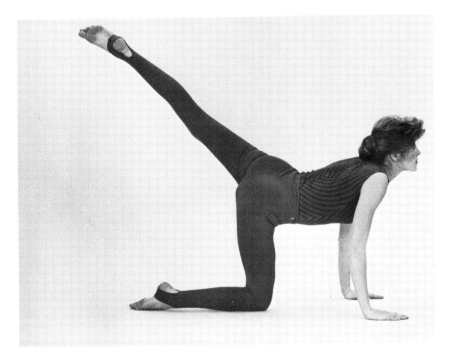

Kick left.

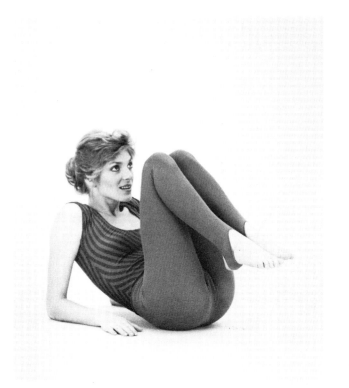

Tuck.

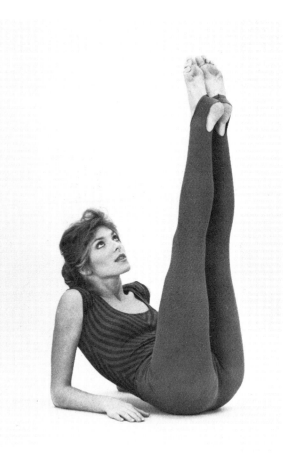

Extend up.

INNER THIGH KICK

Good for inner thighs. Sit resting back on your arms, knees bent and tucked in to your chest, toes pointed. Kick the legs up and straighten. Stretch the legs apart and bring them together. Repeat sequence.

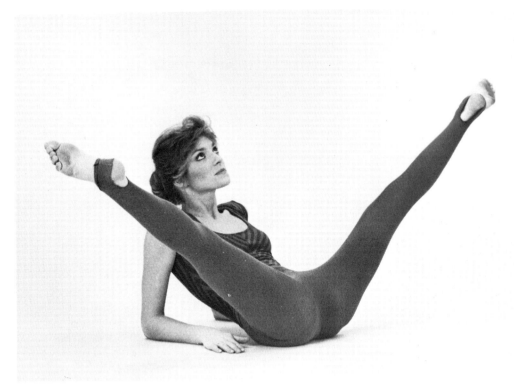

Stretch apart.

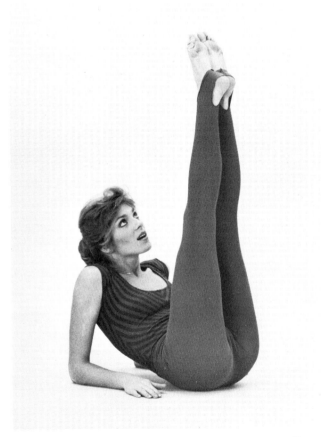

Bring together.

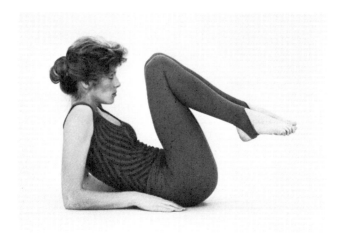

Starting position.

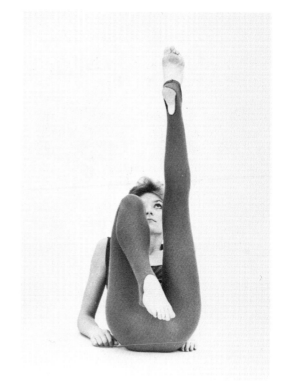

Kick left.

WHIP KICK

Lie down with torso slightly raised, leaning back on the forearms. Tuck both legs in to the chest. Kick the left leg straight up. While rotating on the left hip, kick the right leg out at a 45-degree angle and tuck the left leg. Continue rolling on the hip, kicking the left leg down to the floor and tucking the right leg. Return to the center, alternating kicks, and repeat the sequence to the other side.

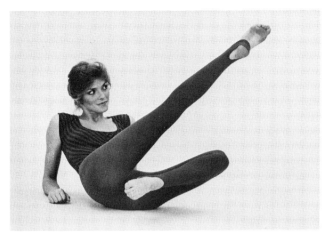

Kick right.

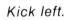

Kick left.

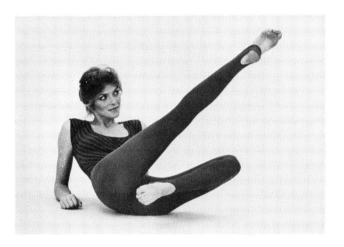

Returning to center, kick right.

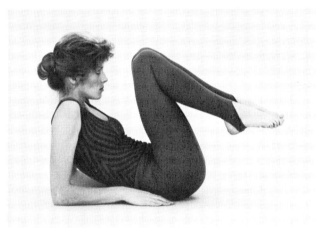

Finish.

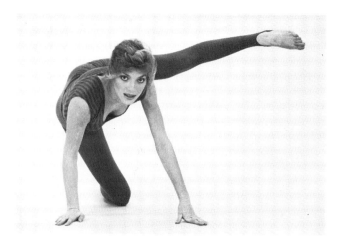

Leg out.

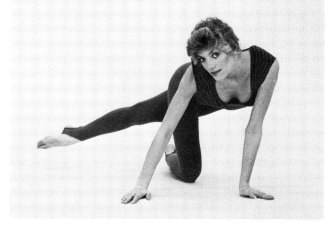

Cross back.

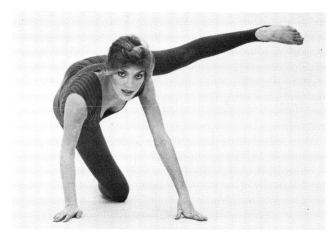

Swing out.

CROSS LEG SWING

Rest your hands and knees. Lift one leg straight out to the side. Swing the leg back and cross to the opposite side. Repeat the swing movement and then alternate legs.

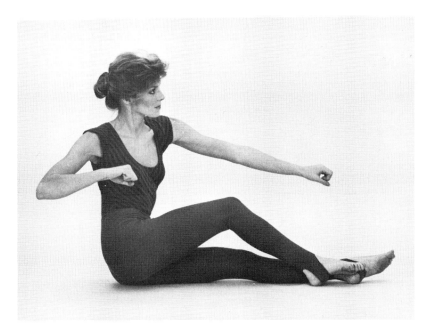

Scoot forward.

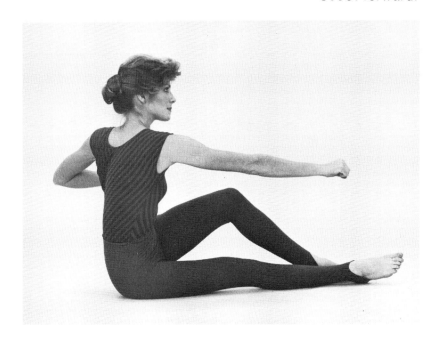

Alternate sides.

WHIP SCOOT

Sit on the floor with legs extended, feet together. Scoot forward from side to side, whipping your arms out front. As you scoot, flex the legs and hips. Repeat, going backward.

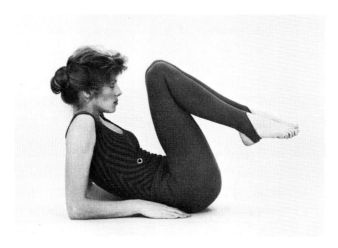

Starting tuck position.

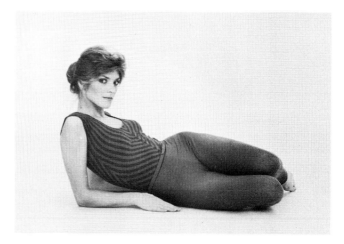

Roll right.

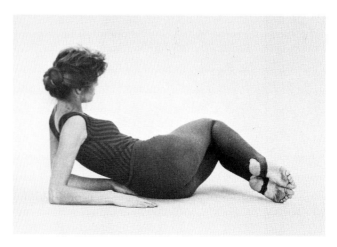

Roll left.

TUCK AND ROLL

Lie down with legs tucked and torso raised, resting back on the forearms. Keeping your knees together, roll to the right and roll to the left.

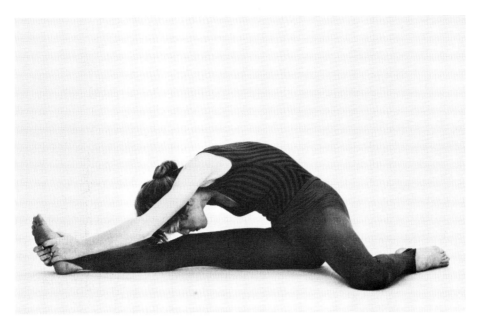

Stretch down.

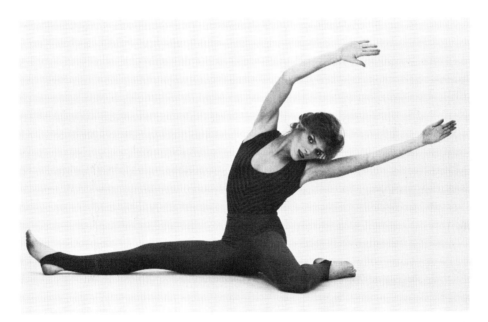

Lift and stretch back.

LEG STRETCH I

Sit down, stretching the right leg in front and tucking the left leg in back. Try to clasp both hands as close to the right ankle as possible. Gently stretch down. Then lift the torso, twisting to the left and stretching back with arms overhead. Repeat the movement to the other side.

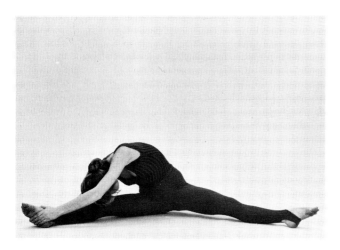

Stretch right.

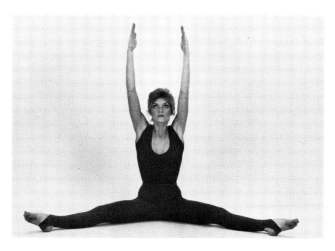

Return to center, arms overhead.

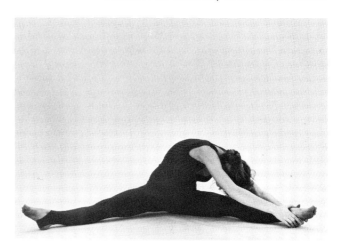

Stretch left.

LEG STRETCH II

Extend the legs out straight to the side as far as possible, toes pointed and feet turned out. Twisting to the right, clasp both hands as close to the right ankle as possible. Gently stretch. Return to the center and repeat the stretch to the other leg.

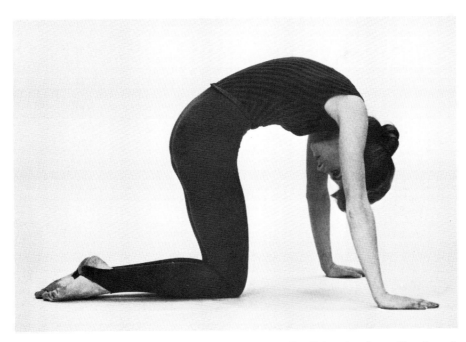

Roll back; drop the head.

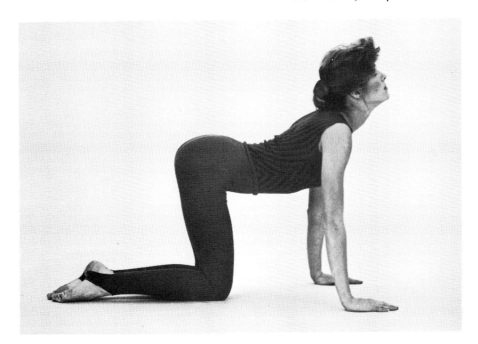

Arch the back; lift the chin.

THE CAT

Resting on palms and knees, round the back,
pulling the shoulders forward and bending
the head down. Then lift the chin up while
arching back. Repeat the movement.

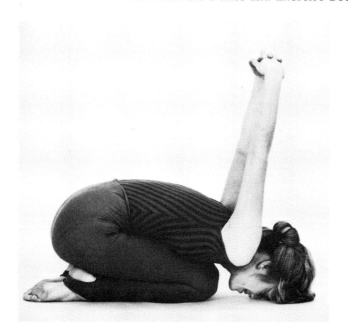

Starting position.

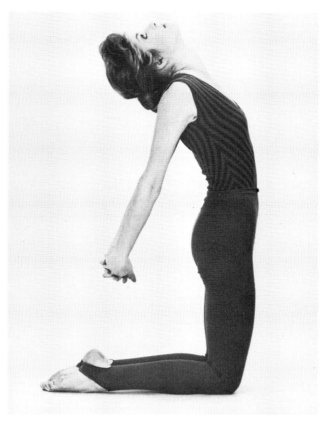

Lift up and stretch back.

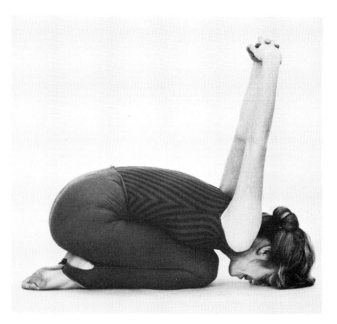

Return to the original position.

YOGA STRETCH I

Start in the tucked position, forehead to the floor and arms stretched straight overhead with hands clasped. Lift up from the knees, stretching back as far as you can comfortably go. Return to the starting position. Repeat the sequence.

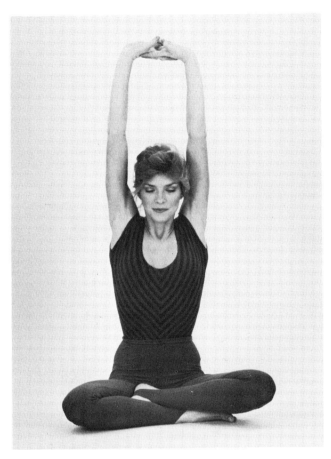

Stretch up, arms overhead.

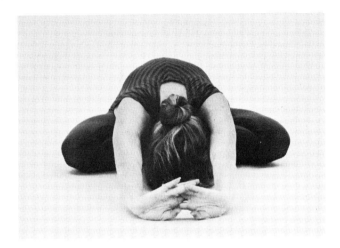

Stretch down, arms in front.

YOGA STRETCH II

Good stress releaser. Sit down with legs crossed in front. With hands flexed, stretch your arms overhead. Bend forward, bringing the forehead to the floor and stretching the arms out front. Repeat the movement.

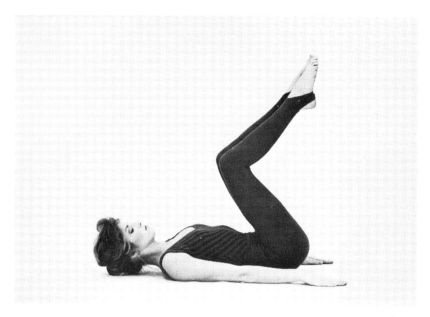

Knees flexed.

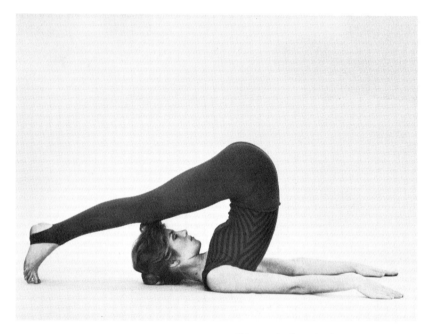

Stretch back, legs straight.

YOGA STRETCH III

Good stress releaser. Lie down and lift your legs up, knees flexed, arms down at your sides for support. Extend the legs and stretch them back over your hands as far as possible, all the way to the floor. Return to the original position.

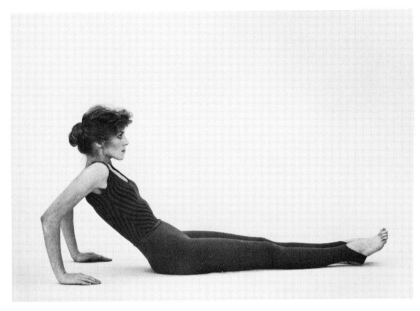

Starting position.

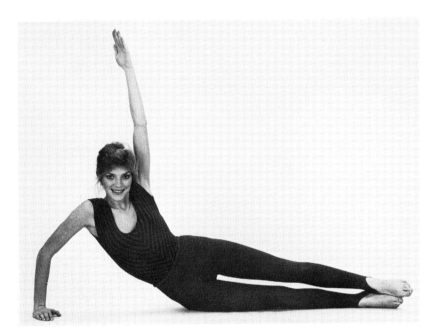

Roll on the hip and raise the opposite arm overhead.

HIP ROLL

Sit down, legs extended and feet together. Rest back on your palms, arms bent. Roll to the right, moving on the right hip, and extend the left arm overhead. Keep the right arm bent. Roll back to the center and repeat to the other side.

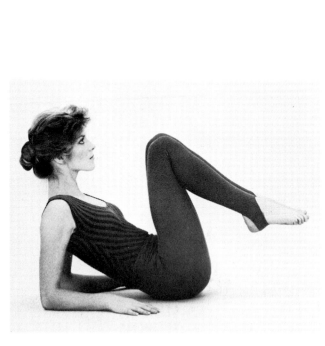

Flex in.

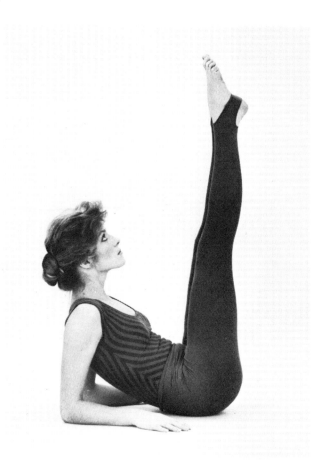

Straighten up.

FLEX STRADDLE KICK

Lie down with torso slightly raised, resting back on the forearms. Flex your legs. Kick the legs straight up. Stretch the legs apart and bring them down to the floor without bending. Bring the legs together.

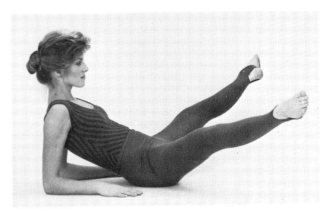

Lower legs to the floor.

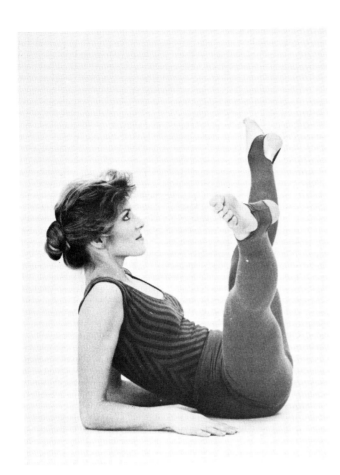

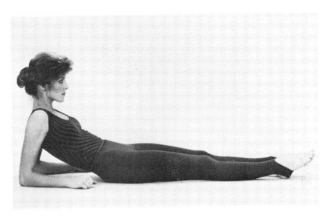

Stretch apart.

Feet together.

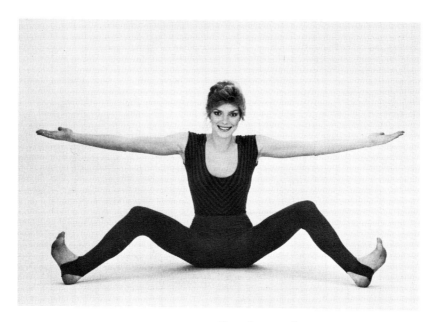

Flex legs, stretch arms to side.

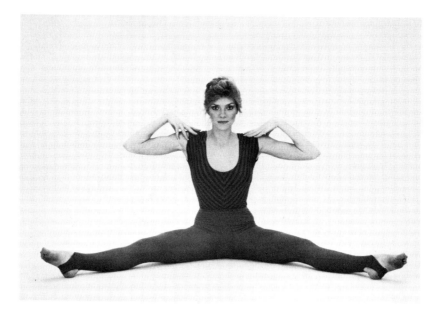

Extend legs, hands to shoulders.

LEG FLEX

Good for inner thighs. Sit with legs and toes flexed to the side, arms straight out to the side. Extend the legs as far out to the side as possible, point your toes, and drop your hands to your shoulders. Flex the knees and toes again, stretching the arms overhead. Extend the legs, again dropping the arms to the shoulders. Remember to keep the back very straight throughout the routine.

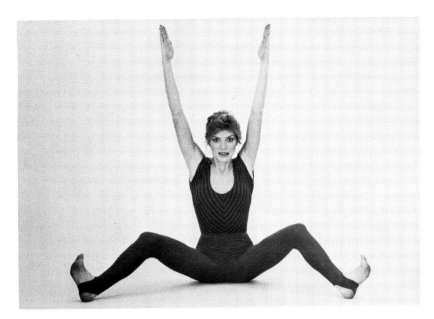

Flex legs, stretch arms overhead.

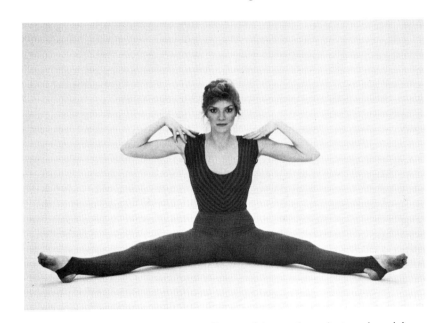

Extend legs, hands to shoulders.

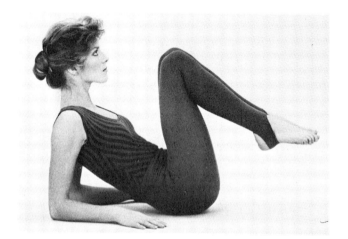

Flex.

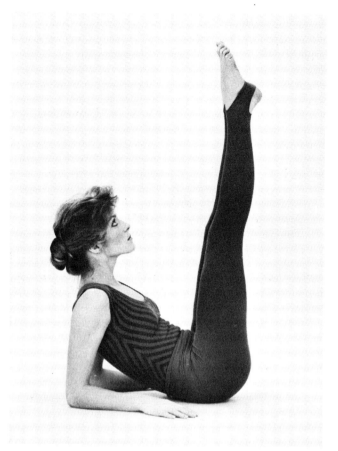

Straight up.

DOUBLE FLEX KICK

Lie down with torso slightly raised, resting back on the forearms. Flex the legs. Lift the legs straight up. Flex the legs again. Lower the legs straight to the floor.

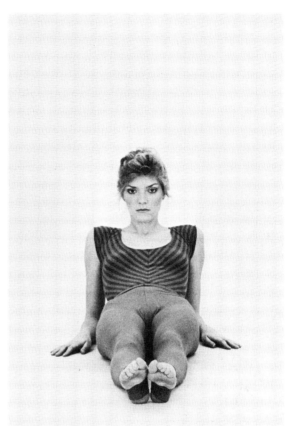

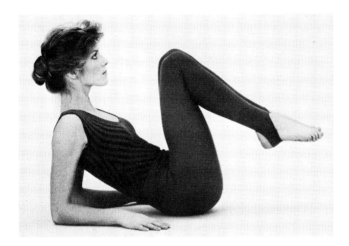

Flex.

Straight down.

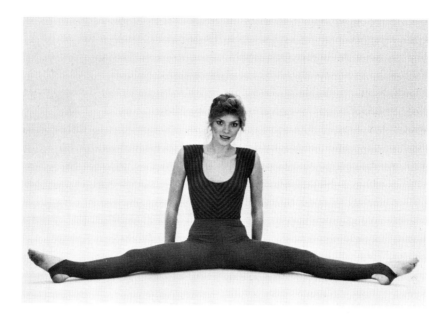

Straddle legs.

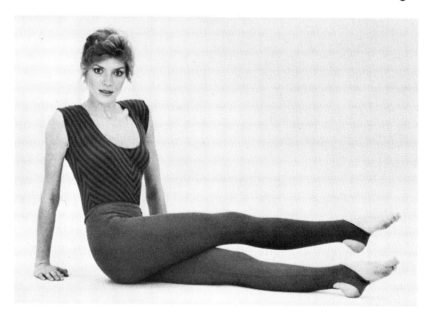

Cross right leg over left.

LEG CROSS

Sit with your legs extended as far to the sides
as possible, toes pointed and back held erect.
Place the arms on the floor behind the legs
and use them as support. Swing the right leg,
crossing over the left leg, which remains flat
on the floor. Return to the original position.
Repeat the sequence, alternating legs.

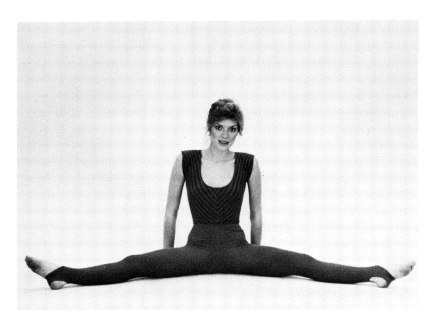

Back to the original position.

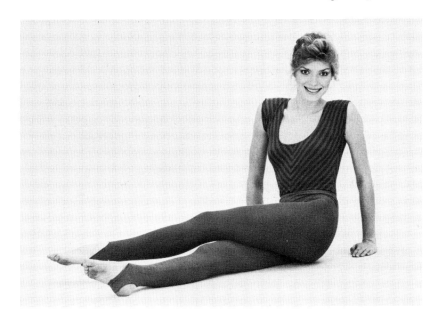

Cross left leg over right.

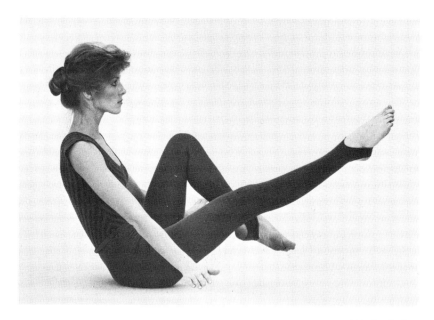

Kick right.

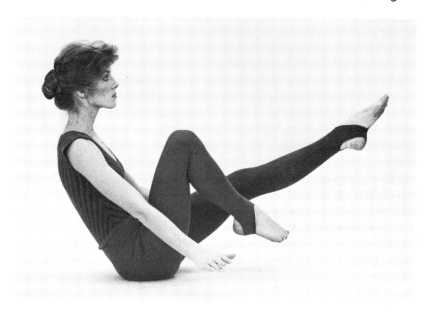

Kick left.

BALANCING KICK

Sit with your knees bent, toes pointed. Lean back slightly, arms out to the side for balance. Kick the right leg straight out. Tuck the right leg in as you kick the left leg straight out. Repeat the kicks, alternating legs.

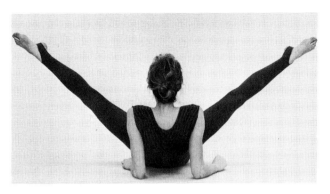

Stretch apart.

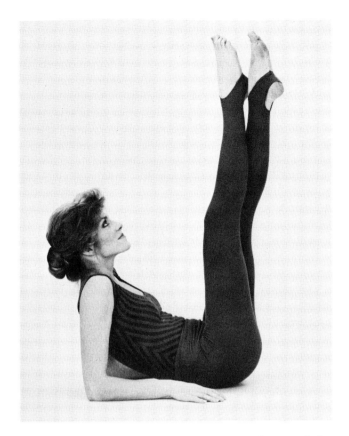

Cross right.

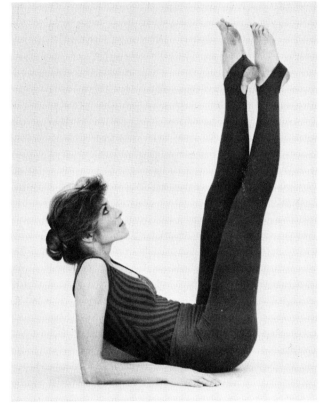

Cross left.

SCISSOR KICK

Lie down with torso raised slightly, resting on your arms for support. With both legs lifted straight up, cross the legs and stretch apart, alternating legs.

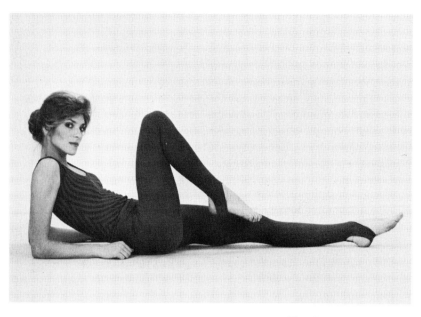

Tuck the right leg.

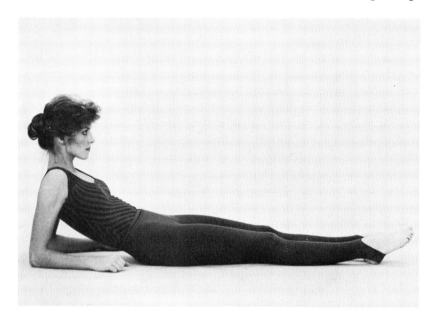

Straighten.

LEG TUCK

Lie down with torso slightly raised, using
your arms for support. Tuck the right leg in
and stretch down. Repeat the movement with
the opposite leg.

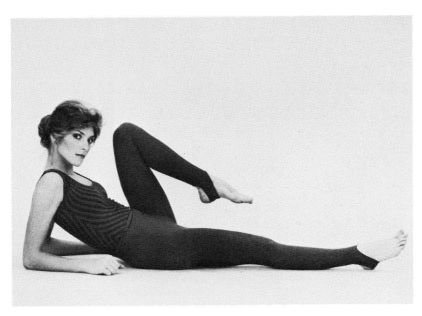

Tuck the left leg.

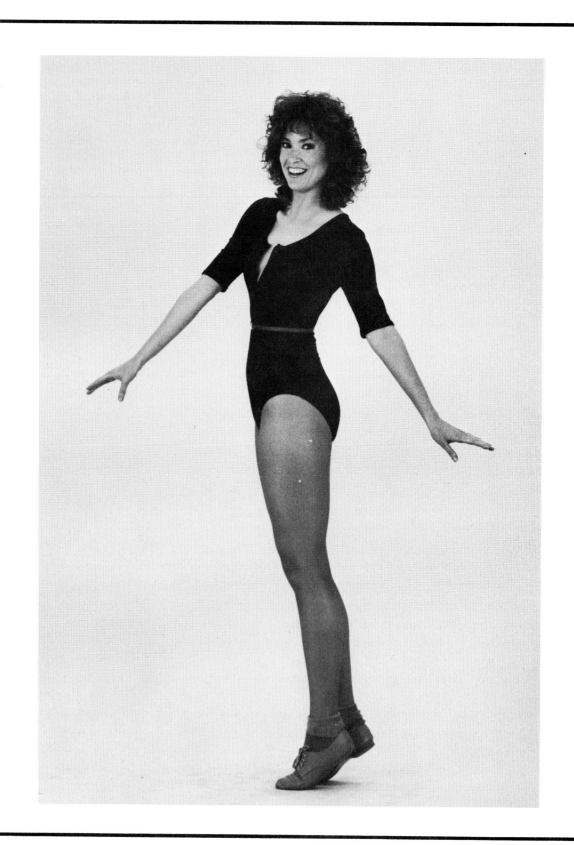

8

Routines

During the routines, if you are out of breath or simply can't keep step, slow down and perhaps do every other beat. You can choreograph the routines to shorter pieces of music or to ones with slower tempos. Beginners should strive for at least 8–10 minutes of continuous aerobic exercise before going to the cooldowns. Remember, though, that only through continued and increased aerobic activity will your entire cardiovascular system and body muscles become stronger. As you progress, simply add five extra minutes of dance routines to your workout until you achieve 40 minutes of continued aerobic activity, which I consider to be advanced level. While I have offered suggested music in my routines, if you don't like or cannot find a particular number, choose an alternate that provides the same tempo.

At the end of the suggested routines that follow is a sample one-hour workout program. While it is designed in its entirety for the advanced aerobic dancer and contains six warm-

ups, four dance routines, and five cool-downs, the workout can be used by beginners as well as intermediates. Simply reduce the number of routines according to your level. Beginners may want to start out with three warm-ups, two dance routines, and two cool-downs. Repeat each exercise eight times. As you progress, keep adding more routines to the workout and increase the number of repetitions for each exercise by eight. For example, intermediates can repeat each exercise 16 times and advanced dancers can repeat up to 32 times. Each warm-up, dance routine, and cool-down has suggested music that will help you select an appropriate tune with the same tempo if you do not have that particular piece of music.

If, during the dance routines you feel the need to stop, simply pause and do some isolated shoulder rolls or side reaches until you catch your breath. Relax, change positions, bounce in place, or take your pulse. Remember, the important thing is to have fun!

Warm-Up Routines

Eye in the Sky —*The Alan Parsons Project*

Reach 16 ×
Side Stretch 16 ×
Toe Touch 16 ×

Bend and Stretch 4 ×
Side Stretch 16 ×
Toe Touch 10 ×

Bend and Stretch 4 ×
Toe Touch 10 ×

Bend and Stretch to end of music

Jump to It —*Aretha Franklin*

Elbow Touch 16 ×
Toe Touch 2 ×
Double Arm Side Stretch 8 ×
Plié 4 ×

Toe Touch 2 ×
Double Arm Side Stretch 8 ×
Plié 4 ×

Toe Touch 1 ×
Double Arm Side Stretch 8 ×
Plié 4 ×

Toe Touch to end of music

Dance Routines

Rock Around the Clock —*Bill Haley and the Comets*

Twist 32 ×

Knee Lift I—2 × on each leg
Knee Slap 4 × on each leg
Side Flick Kick 4 × (right)
Side Flick Kick 4 × (left)

Knee Lift I—2 × on each leg
Knee Slap 4 × on each leg
Side Flick Kick (right) 4 ×
Side Flick Kick (left) 4 ×

Twist 16 ×

Jump Cross 6 ×

Knee Lift I—2 × on each leg
Knee Slap 4 × on each leg
Side Flick Kick (right) 4 ×
Side Flick Kick (left) 4 ×

Twist 16 ×

Knee Lift I—2 × on each leg
Knee Slap 4 × on each leg
Side Flick Kick (right) 4 ×
Side Flick Kick (left) 4 ×

Twist 16 ×

Hop Flick Kick (alternating legs) 12 ×

Knee Lift I—2 × on each leg
Knee Slap 4 × on each leg

Knee Lift I—2 × on each leg
Knee Slap 4 × on each leg
Side Flick Kick (right) 4 ×
Side Flick Kick (left) 4 ×

Twist to end of music

Hound Dog —*Elvis Presley*

Hop Flick Kick (right) 2 ×
Hop Flick Kick (left) 2 ×
Hop Flick Kick (right) 2 ×
Hop Flick Kick (left) 2 ×
Hop Flick Kick (right) 2 ×
Hop Flick Kick (left) 2 ×

Hop Flick Kick (right) 2 ×
Hop Flick Kick (left) 2 ×
Hop Flick Kick (right) 2 ×
Hop Flick Kick (left) 2 ×
Hop Flick Kick (right) 2 ×
Hop Flick Kick (left) 2 ×

Hop Flick Kick (right) 2 ×
Hop Flick Kick (left) 2 ×
Hop Flick Kick (right) 2 ×
Hop Flick Kick (left) 2 ×
Hop Flick Kick (right) 2 ×
Hop Flick Kick (left) 2 ×

Pogo (right) 4 ×
Pogo (left) 4 ×
Pogo (right) 4 ×
Pogo (left) 4 ×
Pogo alternating left and right 8 ×

Hop Flick Kick (right) 2 ×
Hop Flick Kick (left) 2 ×
Hop Flick Kick (right) 2 ×
Hop Flick Kick (left) 2 ×
Hop Flick Kick (right) 2 ×
Hop Flick Kick (left) 2 ×

Pogo (right) 4 ×
Pogo (left) 4 ×
Pogo (right) 4 ×
Pogo (left) 4 ×
Pogo alternating left and right 8 ×

Hop Flick Kick (right) 2 ×
Hop Flick Kick (left) 2 ×
Hop Flick Kick (right) 2 ×
Hop Flick Kick (left) 2 ×
Hop Flick Kick (right) 2 ×
Hop Flick Kick (left) 2 ×

Hop Flick Kick (right) 2 ×
Hop Flick Kick (left) 2 ×
Hop Flick Kick (right) 2 ×
Hop Flick Kick (left) 2 ×
Hop Flick Kick (right) 2 ×
Hop Flick Kick (left) 2 ×

Fame —*Irene Carra*

Jump in Place 4 ×
Clap 2 ×
Jump in Place 4 ×
Clap 2 ×

Jump in Place 4 ×
Clap 2 ×
Jump in Place 4 ×
Clap 2 ×

Side Kick and Cross Over 4 × each leg

Jump in Place 4 ×
Clap 2 ×
Jump in Place 4 ×
Clap 2 ×

Jump in Place 4 ×
Clap 2 ×
Jump in Place 4 ×
Clap 2 ×

Side Kick and Cross Over 4 × each leg

Jump in Place 4 ×

Clap 2 ×
Jump in Place 4 ×
Clap 2 ×

Jump in Place 4 ×
Clap 2 ×
Jump in Place 4 ×
Clap 2 ×

Side Kick and Cross Over 4 × each leg

Side Kick and Cross Over 4 × each leg

Repeat entire routine until music ends.

Cool-Down Routines

Truly —*Lionel Ritchie*

Leg Stretch I (right side) 8 ×
Balancing Sit-Up 8 ×

Leg Cross 16 ×
Balancing Sit-Up 8 ×

Leg Stretch I (left side) 16 ×

Finish standing with arms overhead

The Look of Love —*ABC*

The Cat (hold for 2 counts)

Side Flex Kick (right leg) 8 ×
Side Flex Kick (left leg) 8 ×

Flutter Kick 30 ×

Side Flex Kick (right leg) 8 ×
Side Flex Kick (left leg) 8 ×

Flutter Kick 30 ×
The Cat 8 ×

Flutter Kick 30 ×
The Cat 8 ×

Side Flex Kick (right leg) 8 ×
Side Flex Kick (left leg) 8 ×

The Cat 8 ×

I Will Survive —*Gloria Gaynor*

Tuck Stretch Kick (right side) 24 ×
Swing Sit-Up 8 ×

Tuck Stretch Kick (left side) 24 ×
Swing Sit-Up 4 ×

Inner Thigh Kick 15½ ×
Inner Thigh Kick (slower) 7½ ×

Swing Sit-Up 4 ×

Tuck Stretch Kick (right side) 24 ×
Swing Sit-Up 8 ×

Tuck Stretch Kick (left side) 24 ×
Swing Sit-Up 3½ ×

Inner Thigh Kick 15½ ×
Inner Thigh Kick (slower) 7½ ×

Swing Sit-Up 12 ×

ONE-HOUR WORKOUT ROUTINE
(Repeat each exercise 8, 16, 24, or 32 times,
depending upon your level.)

Warm-Up I

Suspicion—*Eddie Rabbitt*

Reach
Relax forward

Side Stretch
Sweep Around
Bend and Stretch

Side Stretch
Sweep Around
Bend and Stretch to end of music

Warm-Up II

Arthur's Theme—*Christopher Cross*

Side Reach
Back Stretch

Plié
Side Stretch Plié
Lunge
Bend and Stretch

Plié
Side Stretch Plié
Lunge
Bend and Stretch to end of music

Warm-Up III

Hard to Say—*Dan Fogelberg*

Reach
Swing Stretch
Feet Flex
Swing Stretch
Toe Touch
Elbow Lift and Swing
Feet Flex
Swing Stretch
Toe Touch
Elbow Lift and Swing to end of music

Warm-Up IV

Sing a Song—*Earth, Wind & Fire*

Forward Lunge
Side Stretch
Plié
Elbow Swing and Side Step
Forward Lunge
Side Stretch
Plié
Elbow Swing and Side Step to end of music

Dance Warm-Up I

Steppin' Out—*Kool & The Gang*

Forward Lunge
Arm Swing
Knee Lift I

Elbow Swing and Side Step
Knee Lift II

Elbow Swing and Side Step
Knee Lift II

Dance Warm-Up II

What a Fool Believes—*The Doobie Brothers*

Head Roll
Knee Lift I

Forward Bob
Cross Lunge
Forward Bob

Knee Lift I
Forward Bob
Cross Lunge
Forward Bob to end of music

Dance Routine I

You May Be Right—*Billy Joel*

Jump in Place (shake shoulders)
Twist
Hopscotch
Hip Swing with Side Step
Side Flick Kick

Twist
Hopscotch
Hip Swing with Side Step
Side Flick Kick

Dance Routine II

Shake It Up—*The Cars*

Knee Hip
Twist
Jump Cross
Flick Kick Front and Side

Knee Hip
Twist
Jump Cross
Flick Kick Front and Side

Dance Routine III

Start Me Up—*The Rolling Stones*

Toe Touch
Pogo
Toe Touch
Pogo
Side Flick Kick

Toe Touch

Pogo
Toe Touch
Pogo
Side Flick Kick

Dance Routine IV

Mickey—*Toni Basil*

Jump in Place with Arm Swing
Hopscotch
Jump in Place with Arm Swing
Pogo
Knee Slap (both legs)

Jump in Place with Arm Swing
Hopscotch
Jump in Place with Arm Swing
Pogo
Knee Slap (both legs)

Dance Cool-Down I

Up Where We Belong—*Joe Cocker and Jennifer Warnes*

Lunge
Back and Leg Stretch
Plié
Leg Stretch I (right side)
Leg Stretch I (left side)

Cool-Down II

Down Under—*Men at Work*

Side Leg Kick (right side)
Swing Sit-Up
Side Leg Kick (left side)
Swing Sit-Up
Double Flex Kick

Side Leg Kick (right side)
Swing Sit-Up
Side Leg Kick (left side)
Swing Sit-Up
Double Flex Kick

Cool-Down III

Hit Me with Your Best Shot—*Pat Benetar*

The Cat
Side Flex Kick (both legs)
Cross Leg Swing (both legs)

Side Flex Kick (both legs)
Cross Leg Swing (both legs)

The Cat
Side Flex Kick (both legs)
Cross Leg Swing (both legs)

Cool-Down IV

Let's Dance—*David Bowie*

Flex Straddle Kick

Scissor Kick

Flex Straddle Kick
Scissor Kick

Hip Roll

Cool-Down V

Chariots of Fire—*Vangelis*

Side Leg Kick (both sides)
Rhythmic Sit-Up
Balancing Kick (both sides)
Forward Leg Stretch
Yoga Stretch I
Yoga Stretch II

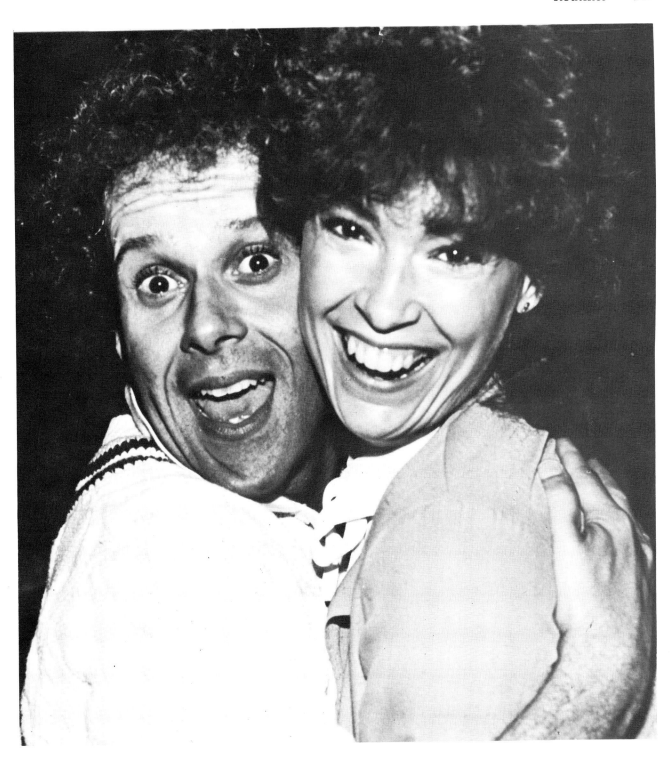

Index